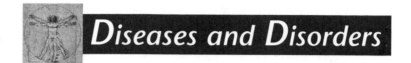

Diseases and Disorders

Hemophilia

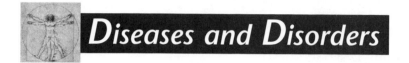
Diseases and Disorders

Hemophilia

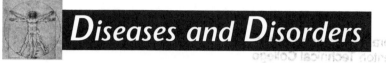

Diseases and Disorders

Hemophilia

by Beverly Britton

LUCENT BOOKS®

THOMSON
™
GALE

San Diego • Detroit • New York • San Francisco • Cleveland
New Haven, Conn. • Waterville, Maine • London • Munich

THOMSON
———————★———————
GALE

© 2003 by Lucent Books. Lucent Books is an imprint of The Gale Group, Inc.,
a division of Thomson Learning, Inc.

Lucent Books® and Thomson Learning™ are trademarks used herein under license.

For more information, contact
Lucent Books
27500 Drake Rd.
Farmington Hills, MI 48331-3535
Or you can visit our Internet site at http://www.gale.com

LIBRARY OF CONGRESS CATALOGING-IN-PUBLICATION DATA
Britton, Beverly. 　　Hemophilia / by Beverly Britton. 　v. cm. — (Diseases and disorders) 　Includes bibliographical references and index. 　Contents: Hemophilia, an ancient disease with a promising future — Understanding hemophilia — Hemophilia throughout history — Diagnosis and treatment — Complications — Living with hemophilia—an accident waiting to happen — The future. 　　ISBN 1-56006-906-6 　1. Hemophilia--Juvenile literature. [1. Hemophilia. 2. Diseases.] I. Title. II. Diseases and disorders series. 　　RC642 .S53 2003 　　616.1'572--dc21 　　　　　　　　　　　　　　　　　　　　　　　　　　　　2002012563

Printed in the United States of America

Table of Contents

"The Most Difficult Puzzles Ever Devised"

C HARLES BEST, ONE of the pioneers in the search for a cure for diabetes, once explained what it is about medical research that intrigued him so. "It's not just the gratification of knowing one is helping people," he confided, "although that probably is a more heroic and selfless motivation. Those feelings may enter in, but truly, what I find best is the feeling of going toe to toe with nature, of trying to solve the most difficult puzzles ever devised. The answers are there somewhere, those keys that will solve the puzzle and make the patient well. But how will those keys be found?"

Since the dawn of civilization, nothing has so puzzled people— and often frightened them, as well—as the onset of illness in a body or mind that had seemed healthy before. A seizure, the inability of a heart to pump, the sudden deterioration of muscle tone in a small child—being unable to reverse such conditions or even to understand why they occur was unspeakably frustrating to healers. Even before there were names for such conditions, even before they were understood at all, each was a reminder of how complex the human body was, and how vulnerable.

While our grappling with understanding diseases has been frustrating at times, it has also provided some of humankind's most heroic accomplishments. Alexander Fleming's accidental discovery in 1928 of a mold that could be turned into penicillin has resulted in the saving of untold millions of lives. The isolation of the enzyme insulin has reversed what was once a death sentence for anyone with diabetes. There have been great strides in combating conditions for which there is not yet a cure, too. Medicines can help AIDS patients live longer, diagnostic tools such as mammography and ultrasounds can help doctors find tumors while they are treatable, and laser surgery techniques have made the most intricate, minute operations routine.

This "toe-to-toe" competition with diseases and disorders is even more remarkable when seen in a historical continuum. An astonishing amount of progress has been made in a very short time. Just two hundred years ago, the existence of germs as a cause of some diseases was unknown. In fact, it was less than 150 years ago that a British surgeon named Joseph Lister had difficulty persuading his fellow doctors that washing their hands before delivering a baby might increase the chances of a healthy delivery (especially if they had just attended to a diseased patient)!

Each book in Lucent's *Diseases and Disorders* series explores a disease or disorder and the knowledge that has been accumulated (or discarded) by doctors through the years. Each book also examines the tools used for pinpointing a diagnosis, as well as the various means that are used to treat or cure a disease. Finally, new ideas are presented—techniques or medicines that may be on the horizon.

Frustration and disappointment are still part of medicine, for not every disease or condition can be cured or prevented. But the limitations of knowledge are being pushed outward constantly; the "most difficult puzzles ever devised" are finding challengers every day.

Hemophilia—An Ancient Disease with a Promising Future

HEMOPHILIA IS THE oldest recorded hereditary bleeding disease. From biblical times to the 1800s, people knew the bleeding disorder existed mainly in males; they just did not know what caused it or how to treat it. It was centuries before it was known that hemophiliacs lacked an essential blood protein needed to make blood clot. The course of hemophilia through the years extends from trial- and-error treatments to some of the most exciting discoveries of this past century.

These steps forward came at a price for the hemophilia community in the 1980s, when 50 percent of hemophiliacs became infected with human immunodeficiency virus (HIV), the virus that leads to full-blown AIDS. This disaster was brought on when patients were treated with clotting factors extracted from human blood that was contaminated with HIV. Suddenly, all the promise and hope of the golden era of hemophilia treatment turned to tragedy as more than four thousand of the hemophilia population in the United States died from AIDS. As recently as 1998, it was estimated there were three hundred deaths a year among AIDS-infected hemophilia patients.

Hemophiliacs living in poorer countries face challenges that are different from those in industrialized nations as they cope with the disease. Eighty percent of hemophiliacs around the world have no available treatment even today, and suffer the pain, joint deformities, and shortened life span that accompany untreated hemophilia. Their plight is no better than those who lived with hemophilia hundreds of years ago.

For those in industrialized countries with access to modern treatment, younger patients fare much better than their fathers or grandfathers ever did as a result of better therapy. Newer treatments have made a difference over time for generations of hemophiliacs. Two generations ago, a hemophiliac would have been treated before newer clotting factors were developed. As a child, the sufferer would have spent a lot of time in the hospital. Hemophiliacs of that era suffered severe pain and developed arthritis from uncontrolled bleeding episodes in the joints. Patients were probably in their mid-forties before at-home treatment for bleeding became available. In adulthood, hemophiliacs of two generations ago might be confined to a wheelchair and unable to work.

The next generation of hemophiliacs began treatment when newer products were available. Hemophiliacs of this generation grew up administering their own treatment at home after each bleed. As adults, their state of health permitted working full-time, marrying, having children, and achieving independence. Side effects of the illness in this generation were mainly mild knee or hip arthritis.

The present generation has benefited from all the newer technology. These hemophiliacs treat themselves at home with preventive measures to keep bleeds from occurring, and lead busy lives with few or no complications. Current hemophiliacs play sports, go to summer camps, and are impossible to distinguish from other people without the disease. The lifestyle of the hemophiliac at the beginning of the twenty-first century is near normal, thanks to the latest treatments.

More progress has occurred in the disease of hemophilia in the last thirty years than in all previous centuries. Kathy Bosma, a nurse who works with hemophilia patients, says, "Just in my lifetime, the change in treatment has been pretty astounding. We've really come a long way."[1] The next few years promise some very exciting discoveries in hemophilia treatment including the very real possibility of a cure for a disease that currently lasts for the lifetime of the sufferer.

Chapter 1

Understanding Hemophilia

HEMOPHILIA IS CAUSED by the body's inability to make a protein necessary for blood to clot. When a person with hemophilia is injured, the blood clots very slowly or sometimes does not clot at all. This can lead to excessive bruising and painful bleeding inside the body into muscles, joints, or body cavities. The word *hemophilia* literally describes the disease: "hemo" means blood and "philia" means having a tendency toward something. Therefore, a person with hemophilia has a tendency toward bleeding.

Large bruises, such as this one on a baby's chest, are a painful symptom of hemophilia.

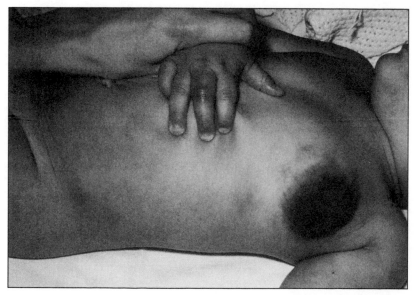

Hemophilia is a rare, genetic disease, which means it is inherited and is passed from one generation to the next. Hemophilia occurs almost exclusively in males and affects only one of every ten thousand. It is a chronic disease, meaning there is currently no cure and the problem lasts throughout the life of the affected person. At present, there is no way to prevent hemophilia, but it can be treated.

Unlike some other inherited diseases, such as sickle cell anemia or cystic fibrosis, hemophilia is not predominant in any particular race, nationality, or socioeconomic group. Hemophilia can be found in people of all races in populations throughout the world and occurs at similar rates among all ethnic and racial groups. Hemophilia is also known to exist in horses and in nine breeds of dogs.

The A and B of Hemophilia

The two most common types of hemophilia are hemophilia A and hemophilia B, also called Christmas disease, since it was named after a young boy, Stephen Christmas, who was the first person identified to have this type of hemophilia. A person with hemophilia will have either A or B, but not both types. These two types of hemophilia account for almost 100 percent of hemophilia cases, although there is a type C hemophilia, which affects both sexes and causes mild bleeding, like nosebleeds, unrelated to trauma (a bodily injury). Other diseases where blood clotting is not normal are not classified as hemophilia. Some of these bleeding diseases are so rare that there are only a few known cases in the world.

Of the two main types, hemophilia A is the most common. Eighty percent of all cases of hemophilia are classified as hemophilia A. Hemophilia A affects about 13,500 Americans. The disease is also called classic hemophilia.

Classic or hemophilia A is caused by a decreased or missing factor in the blood called factor VIII, which is one of the chemicals necessary for effective blood clotting. Factor VIII is manufactured in the liver and circulates in the liquid part of the blood known as the plasma. Varying amounts of factor VIII in the blood determine whether the disease is classified as mild, moderate, or severe. The usual amount of factor VIII in the blood is stated in lab books as

55 to 145 percent of normal. This measurement is based on testing the blood of a large group of people with supposedly normal amounts of the factor. One hundred percent is the average in the tested group, with a range of values from 55 to 145. The test does not directly measure the clotting factor, but measures its functional activity. In mild hemophilia A, the person may have 5 to 50 percent of the normal amount of factor VIII working to clot blood. If only 1 to 5 percent of factor VIII is active, the person's blood clots less well, and he has moderate hemophilia. In severe hemophilia the person has as little as 1 percent or less of factor VIII and is prone to more frequent and severe bleeds.

Hemophilia B, or Christmas disease, has similarities with A but affects fewer people and is caused by a lack of a different clotting factor. In contrast to hemophilia A, which affects one in ten thousand people, hemophilia B is rarer still, affecting only one in forty thousand people. Hemophilia B is responsible for 15 to 20 percent of hemophilia cases. In hemophilia B the missing or defective clotting factor is called factor IX, which, like the factor

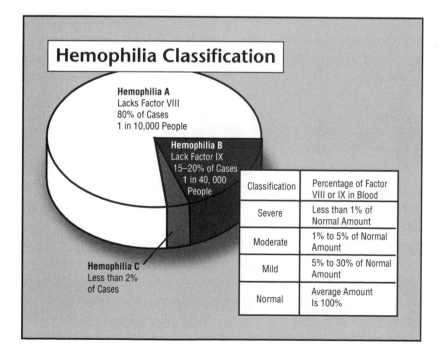

Hemophilia Classification

Hemophilia A
Lacks Factor VIII
80% of Cases
1 in 10,000 People

Hemophilia B
Lack Factor IX
15–20% of Cases
1 in 40, 000 People

Hemophilia C
Less than 2% of Cases

Classification	Percentage of Factor VIII or IX in Blood
Severe	Less than 1% of Normal Amount
Moderate	1% to 5% of Normal Amount
Mild	5% to 30% of Normal Amount
Normal	Average Amount Is 100%

missing in hemophilia A, circulates in the plasma portion of the blood ready to help with blood clotting. Like hemophilia A, not everyone with hemophilia B bleeds with the same intensity, due to varying amounts of factor IX in their blood. Normal percentages for factor IX are 60 to 140, with 100 being the average amount. Mild hemophilia B patients possess 5 to 50 percent of clotting factor IX, moderate cases will have 1 to 5 percent of the clotting factor, and severe cases will have less than 1 percent available to help form a clot. All members of a family with hemophilia tend to have the same amount of clotting factor.

The Family Connection

Hemophilia is a genetic disorder, which means it is passed from one generation to the next. Genes, inside body cells, are responsible for each person's unique characteristics, and determine everything from a person's height and eye color to tendencies toward some illnesses. If a gene is defective or missing, then it can cause an illness such as hemophilia. "One hundred thousand genes carry the instructions to bring a baby to life. The only difference between a baby with hemophilia and a baby without hemophilia is that one gene does not work properly in the hemophilic child,"[2] says Peter Jones, M.D. In addition to hemophilia, there are about four thousand diseases caused by genetic defects.

In hemophilia, there is usually a family history of the disease. Family members carry a defective version of the gene that is necessary to complete a clot that will stop the bleeding until the body can repair the damaged area.

To comprehend how hemophilia is passed from one generation to the next, it is necessary to understand chromosomes. All humans have twenty-three pairs of chromosomes, which are threadlike chemical structures inside cells. Chromosomes carry genes, which contain the code for inherited traits. Half of each chromosome pair is inherited from a person's mother and half from the father.

One pair of chromosomes is responsible for determining a person's sex. If a person receives two X chromosomes, one from the mother and one from the father, to make a pair, a female results (XX). If an X and a Y chromosome are joined, the sex is male (XY).

This is important in hemophilia, since the affected blood clotting genes in hemophilia are on the X chromosome. Because the blood clotting genes reside on the chromosome that determines sex, the disease is called X-linked or sex-linked.

Women can be carriers of hemophilia, meaning they can pass it on to sons without having symptoms themselves. This is true because the genes determining hemophilia are recessive. Genes are either dominant (stronger) or recessive (weaker). In the science of genetics, recessive diseases require two defective genes, one from the mother and one from the father, before the actual disease is present in their child. Hemophilia is carried on the X chromosome, and so if one of a woman's X chromosomes carried the defect, her other normal X chromosome would dominate, canceling out the defective one. Since it is unlikely that a woman would have defective genes on both X chromosomes, women rarely have hemophilia. Since men have only one X chromosome, if they receive a defective X chromosome from their mother, they do not have a second normal X chromosome, capable of producing the missing clotting factor, to counteract the defective one. Because of this, one defective gene is enough to cause hemophilia.

The chances of a son having hemophilia if the mother has a defective gene are 50 percent, or one chance out of two. La Donna Loehrke of North Dakota had the following reaction when informed that her son had hemophilia. "I was upset, mad, unbelieving, and feeling that it was my fault. Although it runs in our family, we thought it would not happen to us."[3] The 50 percent chance is true for every pregnancy a woman has. This means if a carrier woman gives birth to one son who has hemophilia, the next time she gives birth to a son, there is still a 50 percent chance that he will also have hemophilia. An example of this is the family of Ricky Ray, a hemophilia patient from Florida, whose two brothers also have hemophilia.

In a similar way, daughters of carrier women have a 50 percent chance of receiving the faulty gene and becoming carriers. This means any future male children they have also have a 50 percent chance of having hemophilia.

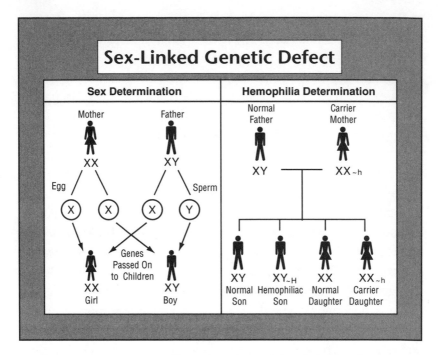

There is only one way that a female could suffer from the disease of hemophilia. If her mother were a carrier and contributed the defective gene and her father had hemophilia, both her X chromosomes would carry the gene for hemophilia and she would have the disease. Not every female born to the family would necessarily have hemophilia, since some females might inherit the mother's normal X chromosome. Therefore, females born to that family would have a one in two chance of having hemophilia.

In one-third of all cases of hemophilia, no family history can be found. In these cases, the disease is caused by spontaneous gene mutation. A mutation is a permanent, unusual change in a gene, which prevents it from performing its task. Hemophilia is actually thought to have originated hundreds of generations ago through gene mutation. Gene mutations can occur at the very beginning of a pregnancy or much later in life in a parent, who can then pass the mutated gene to future offspring. Genes mutate due to aging or exposure to chemicals or radiation. In the case of hemophilia, the change affects the genes that code for factor VIII or factor IX, and becomes a permanent part of the genetic makeup of that person.

To Clot or Not

A person born with hemophilia has inherited a problem with blood clotting. The process of blood clotting is complex, but basically involves three steps. If any of these steps does not work, then the person will bleed longer than normal. In hemophilia, the first two steps occur normally, but the third step of blood clotting is impaired, which prevents the final clot from forming.

The first step occurs when a person receives an injury that allows blood to escape from an artery or a vein. The blood vessel immediately constricts (becomes smaller) to decrease the flow of blood.

The second event involves platelets, one of the three types of cells circulating in the blood. The other two types of cells are red blood cells and white blood cells, but only platelets contribute to clotting. Platelets migrate to the opening in the vessel and clump together in an attempt to plug the leaking blood. Their purpose is to form a soft clot until a more permanent one can be made. This step takes about one minute. Platelets also have a role in the final clot when protein factors are added to them to make a stronger, permanent clot.

Step three of the clotting process is the most complex because it involves twelve clotting factors, identified by roman numerals. These protein factors work together to form the final clot of fibrin, which is a tangle of threads forming a net over the platelets to hold them firmly against the open wound. This step of forming the final clot includes factor VIII and factor IX and a few clotting factors found in surrounding tissue. The process of forming a final clot is often referred to as a clotting cascade because each factor or chemical stimulates the next factor in a series of events that results in a clot. This can take from two to six minutes. The clotting cascade is similar to setting a row of dominos on end and pushing the first one in line, which topples the second one, and so on until all dominos react to that initial push. If any one domino fails to topple, all dominos after it remain standing. In blood clotting, the final clot depends on all the clotting factors being present and working. If any are missing, the process of forming a clot comes to a halt, which is what happens in hemophilia. The missing or defective factor VIII or IX stops the progression of the clotting cascade.

The Symptoms of Hemophilia

Since the clotting cascade is incomplete in a hemophiliac, bleeding can range from a minor to a very serious event. The main problem is that the person with hemophilia will bleed longer than normal and needs close attention to assure the bleeding is controlled.

Contrary to common belief, hemophiliacs will not bleed to death from a skin cut. Hemophiliacs take longer to form a clot than the average person, but their bleeding is not faster. It is slow, steady, and continuous, but it does not gush from the wound. Therefore, normal first aid measures will control most external bleeds.

Internal bleeding is far more serious than minor cuts on the skin's surface, since it is less obvious and may go unnoticed. Internal bleeding can be caused by injury or can occur spontaneously. Most hemophiliacs learn to recognize signs of an internal bleed. When the bleeding is in a joint, the first symptom may be a prickly or bubbly sensation. As the bleeding continues, it can cause severe pain, particularly if it is bleeding into a rigid space like a joint and is not controlled. Later symptoms are numbness, swelling, or tightness.

Bleeding into joints is the most common type of internal bleeding. Treatment needs to be started in the first four hours to prevent pain from the accumulation of blood. Over a period of time, joint bleeds can lead to arthritis and permanent joint damage. Peter Green, a lecturer in molecular genetics, described his experience with joint bleeds in a medical journal. "I had my first hemorrhage into an ankle joint before I could walk, and as childhood progressed, more of my joints succumbed to their first bleed. Every bleed into a joint was, at that time, untreatable and took its course, subsiding over 3 to 10 days. I missed a great deal of school because of my disease, and spent many days in hospital."[4]

Muscle bleeding can also happen spontaneously or following an injury. Bleeding into muscles, if not controlled, causes swelling, which has the potential for damaging nerves and blood vessels by pressing on them. This leads to paralysis or permanent muscle damage if the bleeding is not treated promptly.

Normal Clotting Compared to Hemophilia

Time Elapsed	Injury	Immediately	1 Minute	2–6 Minutes
Normal Blood Clot	Bleeding Starts	Vessels Constrict	Platelet Plug	Fibrin Clot
Hemophilia	Bleeding Starts	Vessels Constrict	Incomplete Platelet Plug	Incomplete Formation of Fibrin Clot

Signs of Bleeding in Other Body Parts

Other signs of bleeding include bruises, blood in the urine or bowels, nosebleeds, bleeding inside the head, and neck and throat hemorrhages. Both children and adults with hemophilia bruise easily, but it is rarely a problem. Bleeding into the brain, however, is very serious and can result in death. Often symptoms are not apparent until several days after the injury. Signs of a brain hemorrhage include changes in level of consciousness, head-aches, or nausea and vomiting. David Dupuy of Massachusetts, says,

> David [his son] fell and hit his head at the same time our daughter had the flu. The bump went down quickly and we thought he was OK. Alicia had experienced severe headaches with her flu, and soon David also had headaches. We thought he had the flu, too. After a week, he still had headaches and became very dizzy whenever he sat up. We had him tested, and cranial exams showed he had slight bleeding against the brain.[5]

When a person with hemophilia has a head injury, it is a serious event and treatment measures begin immediately to avoid a brain hemorrhage.

Neck and throat bleeding are also serious because the swelling that results from accumulation of blood can press on the trachea (airway) and interfere with breathing. Any swelling in the neck area of a hemophiliac is investigated as soon as possible for cause.

Signs of Hemophilia by Age

The ages at which symptoms first occur in a hemophiliac are a clue to the severity of the disease. When a child is born with severe hemophilia, defined as less than 1 percent of clotting factor, the symptoms most often occur during the first eighteen months of life. It is rare for a spontaneous bleed to occur in an infant who is not walking or crawling—most bleeds follow trauma (bodily injury) or invasive procedures. Following birth, events such as routine injections or circumcision, a common surgical procedure performed on males, can initiate bleeding episodes. Once a baby starts walking, bleeding may occur following a minor injury. Jill

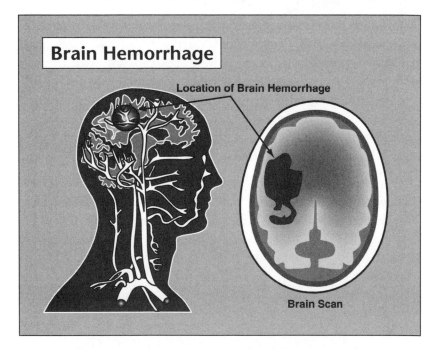

Brain Hemorrhage

Location of Brain Hemorrhage

Brain Scan

and Ric Lathrop of Wisconsin noticed bruising on their infant son, Sam. "Most photographs of Sam from 9 months to 14 months show him with bruises of various shades of yellow, green, and purple."[6]

Toddlers often fall, and bleeding from the lips and tongue is common since these areas contain many blood vessels and bleed easily. Nathan Lambing had this type of injury. His father, Eric, said, "When he was learning to walk, he fell and put his teeth through his upper lip, causing a bleed."[7] About the age of two or three, painful bleeding into muscles or joints following trauma is seen. Those with severe hemophilia bleed into joints, muscles, and other tissues with slight injury or even no obvious injury. They also hemorrhage following surgery or dental extractions. They may have as many as one serious bleed per week.

Moderate hemophiliacs have lengthy bleeds after minor injuries as well as surgery or dental work. Moderate bleeders average a bleed every month.

In milder cases of hemophilia, the first serious bleed may not happen until the child has dental work, surgery, or a more serious accident. Sharon Whiddon of Pennsylvania relates this incident about her son's first bleed. "George's first bleed and subsequent diagnosis happened when he was 15, following wisdom tooth surgery. Before that we had no idea."[8] In some cases of mild hemophilia, the disease is not diagnosed until adulthood. The average number of bleeds per year for mild cases is zero to one. Although the number of times the mild hemophiliac bleeds is no more than many other people experience, the difference remains in the difficulty of controlling the bleeding in a hemophiliac.

Knowledge about blood clotting, symptoms, and patterns of inheritance is essential to a full understanding of hemophilia. Patients are often the experts in the disease, since they live with the effects daily. Peter Green discovered at a young age that he was more knowledgeable than some in the medical field. "'So how long have you had this bad blood?' I was asked as I registered with a new family doctor at the age of 13. I patiently explained that since haemophilia was an inherited disease, I had, of course, had it since birth; my mother was a carrier and her father also had the disease. That many doctors have never heard of Christmas disease [hemophilia B] . . . is surprising but not uncommon." [9]

As Peter Green discovered, many medical professionals, in addition to nonmedical people, do not have full understanding of the disease of hemophilia. Because hemophilia is rare, and genetics and blood clotting are difficult topics for most people to comprehend, a commitment to understanding the disease is the only way for those involved with the care of hemophiliacs to cope. This same principle of commitment to understanding is important for medical personnel and for those interested in learning about the disease. Fortunately, today there is a lot of information available about hemophilia. This has not always been true, because the history of hemophilia leading to the discovery of its causes was long and difficult.

Chapter 2

Hemophilia Throughout History

Although the science of genetics was centuries away, early writers and scientists suspected a family connection to serious bleeding problems. Despite this and other ancient references to the disease dating back almost two thousand years, it has taken many centuries for full understanding to occur. While the hereditary component was recognized, the cause of the problem was thought to be weak blood vessels, not missing clotting factors, as is known today. Understanding of how blood clots did not occur until the 1960s, and the disorder was not called hemophilia until 1828, when a physician named Frederick Hopff, studying at the University of Zurich, gave the disease its current name.

An early reference to the bleeding disorder occurred in the second century A.D. when Jewish writings in the Talmud advised parents to refrain from having a male child circumcised if two previous males in the family had died from bleeding following the procedure. One thousand years later, a Jewish physician recognized the bleeding condition to be hereditary from the mother's side of the family. He advised against circumcising any male children of the same mother when previous male infants had died from bleeding, even if the children had different fathers.

An Arabian physician who lived in Spain, named Albucasis (935–1013), is considered by historians of hemophilia to be one of the key people in the history of the disease. Albucasis was a surgeon

25

who also contributed to the entire field of medicine. His written description of the disease was considered thorough and was the first account of hemophilia by a physician. He, like others, described a family where males died from bleeding problems.

In America, an early reference to hemophilia came in 1803, when Dr. John Conrad Otto of Philadelphia traced a hemorrhagic condition through three generations of a family to a woman who lived near Plymouth, New Hampshire, in 1720. Conrad also recognized that the disease was passed from generation to generation by the mother. His published account of the disease in one family was the first description of hemophilia in America. His observations were recorded in the *Medical Repository*, America's first scientific journal. He wrote:

> About seventy or eighty years ago a woman by the name of Smith . . . transmitted the following idiosyncrasy to her descendants. . . . If the least scratch is made on the skin of some of them, as mortal a hemorrhage will eventually ensue as if the largest wound is inflicted. . . . It is a surprising circumstance that the males only are subject to this strange affection, and that all of them are not liable to it. . . . Although the females are exempt, they are still capable of transmitting it to their male children.[10]

Gregor Mendel and His Peas

In the mid-1800s, Gregor Mendel (1822–1884) made a discovery seemingly unconnected to hemophilia, but which became important in the later understanding of the disease. Mendel, an Austrian monk trained in physics, discovered the basic principles of genetics through his work with plants. He was not a well-known scientist of his day, and he worked alone to discover patterns of inheritance.

As a young boy, Mendel was an excellent student and loved nature, but his parents were poor farmers unable to pay for a university education. So, as a way to continue his education, he entered an Augustinian monastery, where he taught natural science to high school students and bred plants and animals.

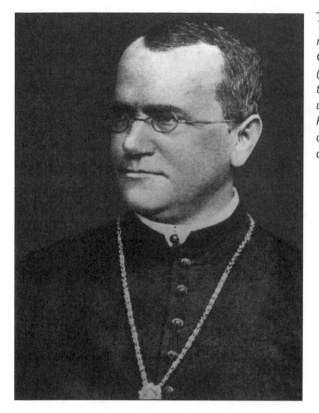

The genetic plant research done by Gregor Mendel (pictured) paved the way to understanding hemophilia and other hereditary diseases.

At the time of Mendel's work, a common theory was that plants obtained their characteristics through the influence of the environment. On one of his daily walks, Mendel discovered a plant that looked different from others of that variety. He transplanted it next to a more typical plant to see what would happen and found that instead of the plant's characteristics being influenced by the environment, the offspring retained the traits of the parent plants. This gave him the idea of heredity.

Mendel began growing sweet peas, and over a period of seven years observed how characteristics of mature plants, like color patterns, passed from generation to generation. He counted the actual ratio of colors in each new plant as a way to predict what future plants would look like. Mendel referred to the parts responsible for inheritance as "factors"; today we call them genes. He recognized that the new plants were receiving half of their characteristics from each parent plant, and he also discovered the concept of dominant (stronger) characteristics. Although other scientists noticed that certain traits pass from animals and plants to their offspring, Mendel was the first to document his results using statistics, and to publish his findings. Unfortunately, his work was published in a local, little-read scientific journal, so it was not until 1900, sixteen years after his death, that scientists discovered his publication. This rediscovery of his principles laid the foundation for modern genetics and its application to humans as well as to plants. Without Gregor Mendel's scientific writings on patterns of inheritance, much of the progress made concerning hemophilia, which occurred in the twentieth century, would have been impossible. Unfortunately, the human application of his principles came too late to explain the appearance of hemophilia in the royal families of Europe.

The Disease of Royalty

The family connection seen in hemophilia received the most publicity during the reign of Queen Victoria of England (1837–1901). Her eighth child, Leopold, had hemophilia and suffered hemorrhages that occurred as often as once a month. Queen Victoria was very protective of Leopold, allowing him few normal activities during his childhood for fear of causing a hemorrhage. Despite the protection given him, he died at the age of thirty-one from a brain hemorrhage after a minor fall. Prior to Leopold's hemophilia, there was no known history of the disease in Queen Victoria's family, leading many historians to believe that Queen Victoria passed the disease because of spontaneous gene mutation. At the time, it was commonly believed the hemophilia in Queen Victoria's family was the result of a curse. Leopold's condition received much attention when it was reported in the *British Medical Journal* in 1868. Queen Victoria herself left a written account of her son's battle with hemophilia in correspondence with her prime minister, Benjamin Disraeli.

Of Queen Victoria's nine children, only three inherited the gene for hemophilia—Leopold, who had the disease, and Alice and Beatrice, who were carriers. Alice and Beatrice passed the defective gene to some of their daughters, who became carriers, who then passed the gene to their sons who had the disease. Beatrice married into the royal family in Spain, and brought the disease of hemophilia to that monarchy. Beatrice's daughter was a carrier and passed the disease of hemophilia to two of her three sons, who both died in young adulthood. Queen Victoria wrote about the family illness, "Our whole family seems persecuted by this awful disease, the worst I know."[11]

One of Alice's daughters, Alexandra, married Nicholas II, a Russian czar of the Romanov family, thus introducing the gene for hemophilia into another royal line. Empress Alexandra gave birth to four girls, and a son, Prince Alexis, who had severe hemophilia. Alexis bruised easily, and one of his knees was permanently damaged from episodes of joint bleeding. A Russian Siberian monk named Rasputin gained great favor in the royal

The young czar Alexis Romanov (seated) suffered from hemophilia, a common disease of royal families until the early twentieth century.

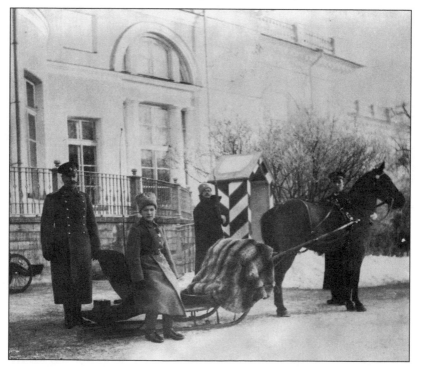

court by treating Alexis with hypnosis to relieve his pain from joint bleeds and also to control some of his bleeding episodes. It is thought that the amount of attention paid to Alexis's illness by his parents, particularly his mother, drew attention away from political problems in Russia in the early 1900s. This may have contributed to the Russian Revolution and the overthrowing of the czar's government in 1917 by the Bolsheviks, who set up a Communist regime. The Bolsheviks murdered the Russian royal family, including fourteen-year-old Alexis and his four sisters, who ranged in age from seventeen to twenty-five.

The current royal family in England descended from Queen Victoria's son, Edward VIII, who did not have hemophilia. The daughter of Beatrice also carried the gene for hemophilia, but gave birth to male children only. Two of her three sons had hemophilia, but only one lived past twenty and he died while a young adult. Irene, one of the daughters of Alice, was also a carrier. She produced two sons, both with hemophilia. One died as a small child, and the other lived into adulthood but did not inherit a throne. Alexandra of Russia, the final carrier of hemophilia and also a daughter of Alice, was murdered in 1918 along with her husband, Nicholas, Alexis, the son who had hemophilia, and their four young daughters who had not married. Thus, the European royal line of hemophilia no longer exists. The disappearance of hemophilia in the European royal families demonstrates the deadliness of hemophilia before modern treatment, since many of the royals died from hemorrhages, which are treatable today.

Christmas Disease

The knowledge of hemophilia advanced in the mid-1900s with the discovery of another form of hemophilia called Christmas disease. Christmas disease is an alternate name for hemophilia B, named for a ten-year-old British boy, Stephen Christmas, who was the first recognized with this type of hemophilia. In 1952, R.A. Biggs, A.S. Douglas of Oxford University and Dr. Mcfarlane, a hematologist, published a paper describing Stephen Christmas's disease as different from hemophilia A, which before that time was thought to be the only type of hemophilia. They based their finding on previous work by a doctor in Argentina.

In 1944, Dr. Pavlosky, the doctor in Argentina, performed a lab test in which he mixed the blood of two hemophiliacs. To his surprise, the blood of each hemophiliac, when mixed with the other blood, caused clotting. At the time, there was no explanation for the phenomenon. Biggs, Douglas, and Mcfarlane used Dr. Pavlosky's discovery eight years later when they were trying to solve the mystery of Stephen Christmas's bleeding disorder. Their work identified two types of hemophilia and recognized that the cause of each was different. Those patients with hemophilia A still had factor IX, the clotting factor for hemophilia B, and hemophilia B patients, while missing the clotting factor for their disease, still had the clotting factor for A. This explains why Dr. Pavlosky achieved clotting when he mixed the two types of blood together. They called the new hemophilia Christmas disease (after their patient), or hemophilia B. It was not until the 1960s that the clotting factors were identified and named, including factor VIII, responsible for hemophilia A, and factor IX, responsible for hemophilia B.

The History of Hemophilia Treatments

While scientists throughout history were attempting to understand hemophilia, many treatments were tried in desperation. Patients were subjected to everything from magic spells to superstitious incantations.

An early treatment for bleeding in the Middle East involved applying ashes to external wounds to stop bleeding. This treatment went along with the culture's reliance on plants, herbs, and nature to cure or relieve conditions.

The use of ice, rest, and splints was also an early treatment and continued to be used until around 1940 for any type of bleeding episode. Kathy Bosma, nurse coordinator at the Comprehensive Center for Bleeding Disorders at Michigan State University, says,

> When I talk to my adult patients, they remember when they were kids spending weeks or months in bed. The idea was that keeping them in bed would decrease their activity, and this

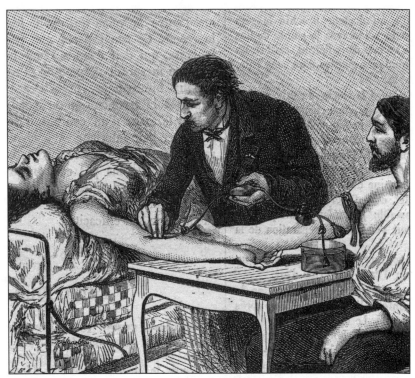

A Victorian woman receives one of the first blood transfusions from a donor.

would minimize the bleeding. They spent a great deal of childhood in bed packed in ice. The ice helped manage the pain and constrict blood vessels, which slows bleeding. Without factor [either factor VIII or factor IX], many of these patients now have terrible joints due to chronic bleeding. [12]

Actually, ice, rest, and splints are still used today, but only for external bleeding or, in the case of splints, for rest of a joint damaged by internal bleeding, not as a way to stop bleeding. Since the most dangerous bleeding is internal, this offered limited help.

Blood transfusions were the first treatment for internal bleeding that actually contained some of the missing clotting factors that are an essential part of modern treatment. Blood transfusions involve removing a pint of blood from a donor and giving it to a patient through a needle placed in a vein. The first blood transfusion given to treat hemophilia was performed in 1840 by a surgeon in London, who administered it to a young man who bled profusely following surgery. The physician reported the case in the British medical journal, *Lancet*. However, at the time, most doctors knew nothing about clotting factors in blood, the different blood types, or even the technique for administering blood, so were unwilling to try the treatment.

It was not until the 1930s that blood transfusions as a method of treatment became popular. The discovery just before 1920 that the cause of hemophilia was a problem of blood clotting and not weak blood vessels encouraged doctors to use whole blood to treat hemophiliacs after they had suffered a serious bleed. Whole blood contains red blood cells, white blood cells, platelets, and plasma plus some of the clotting factors and must be matched to a patient's blood type to prevent an adverse reaction. While this saved some lives by replacing lost blood, it was not totally effective in improving clotting because a pint of blood, the usual amount administered in a transfusion, does not contain enough clotting factors to replace all the factors missing in a hemophiliac. Byard Foraker, a patient with hemophilia, described his early treatment. "By the time I was 24, I had been in the hospital 125 to 130 times. When I was young, the only thing they had to treat me with was whole blood. I always had to go to the hospital because they didn't have anything like the treatments they have today." [13]

Also in the 1930s, physicians tried fasting as a treatment. This required patients to go without food for forty-eight hours. One hemophiliac, named Ben Lederman, was a teenager during the 1930s, and remembers that era as a time of "witches' brews." [14] After he listed everything from cod liver oil to brewer's yeast used as treatments in those days, he said with humor, "Fasting for 48 hours was naturally the final prescription for getting a good clot." [15]

Another treatment, which sounded little better than witches' brews, actually showed some promise in helping blood clot. In 1934, R.G. Mcfarlane, a British hematologist (a specialist in diseases of the blood), reported using a topical solution of snake venom to treat bleeding episodes in hemophiliacs. He discovered that snake venom applied to the wound actually hastened blood clotting, but its use was limited to external bleeding.

The 1950s saw the use of fresh plasma from pigs and cows as a treatment. Plasma is the almost clear, liquid part of blood minus the cells, and is the part of blood containing the clotting factors. It does not need to be matched to the patient's blood type as whole blood does. While the treatment sometimes helped, an unfortunate side effect for a few was allergic reactions to the animal products. As with whole blood, plasma did not contain sufficient amounts of clotting factors to be a totally successful treatment. It was not until later that blood products containing concentrated amounts of clotting factors became the treatment of choice.

The Modern Era of Treatment

While some earlier treatments offered limited help, Dr. Judith Pool is credited with making the first major breakthrough in treating hemophilia A with concentrated amounts of factor VIII. Dr. Pool and her associates made the discovery in 1964 and 1965 that when frozen plasma is slowly thawed, it separates into layers. The bottom layer is rich in clotting factor VIII, the factor missing in type A hemophilia. This discovery was important because for the first time, sufficient amounts of the missing clotting factor could be administered without adding a large volume of fluid to the person's circulatory system and putting unnecessary strain on the heart. The new substance was named cryoprecipitate. Unlike giving whole blood transfusions, cryoprecipitate did not need to match a person's specific blood type. Administration required mixing the thawed plasma with a saline solution and giving it to the patient through a needle into a vein. Several of these small bags of cryoprecipitate were sometimes needed to stop the bleeding. George McCoy used this treatment before other methods were developed. "Before clotting concentrates were available, I used cryoprecipitate, which I kept at home in eight individual plastic bags. I would warm them in pans of water, hang them on an IV pole, self-infuse, and keep changing the bags. It was a long, slow, tedious process that took a few hours each time I needed to infuse."[16] The problem with the new treatment was that it sometimes contained viruses from the human donors, which could cause disease in the person receiving it. Despite this risk, the discovery of cryoprecipitate revolutionized the treatment of hemophilia and was considered a miraculous discovery.

The next advancement in treatment was the introduction of freeze-dried factor concentrates. This discovery made it easier for patients to administer clotting factors at home, thus dramatically decreasing the need for frequent trips to the emergency room. The new innovation in treatment was also made from the plasma of blood donors, but was supplied as a freeze-dried powder. This product was more stable than cryoprecipitate, which had to be administered within four hours of thawing, and was available for both types of hemophilia. It came in small glass bottles, and the patient only needed to add sterile water to the powder, mix it, and then administer it using a sterile needle. With the use of freeze-dried factor concentrates, hemophiliacs were able to travel, attend school regularly, hold down jobs, and lead more normal lives.

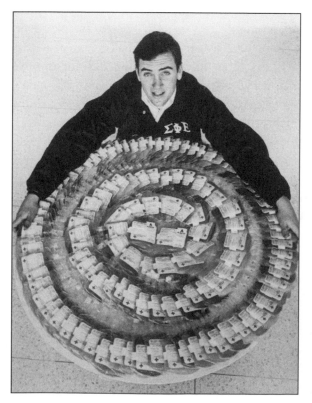

A young hemophiliac encircles the 121 cryoprecipitate packages that stopped his bleeding after a dentist's appointment.

However, like cryoprecipitate, the factor sometimes contained dangerous viruses from the donors.

The New Treatments Become Dangerous

In the 1980s, the treatment, which had offered so much hope to hemophiliacs, suddenly became their worst enemy. The advent of AIDS, a noncurable disease that destroys the body's immune system, had a profound effect on the hemophiliac community. Because AIDS was a new, previously unknown disease, no one suspected that the nation's blood supply would become the vehicle for transmission of a deadly disease to patients requiring blood transfusions or blood products. Unfortunately, the AIDS virus was present in some of the blood used to make cryoprecipitate and the freeze-dried factor concentrates. These products were manufactured from human plasma, and the concentration of clotting factors necessary to stop the bleeding of a hemophiliac came from pooling the blood of multiple donors. Thus, every time a patient received a treatment, he was exposed to the blood of many people. At the time, there was no way to kill the virus in the donated blood. As a result, more than four thousand hemophiliacs contracted AIDS and subsequently died from the very treatment designed to save their lives.

The advent of AIDS caused a frantic search for a safe blood supply for hemophiliacs as well as others. Various methods to kill viruses in blood products were invented. Factors were treated using steam under pressure or dry heat, and very fine filtering devices removed viruses from products. Even pasteurization, first used to purify milk, was used. This method involved heating liquid clotting factor to 140 degrees for ten hours. Another method mixed chemicals with the factors to dissolve the virus's protective coating, thus killing it.

While these methods worked, scientists believed that the safest solution centered on finding a source of treatment not involving the use of human blood. The first step was the discovery in 1984 of the genes that code the human body for the production of factors VIII and IX. Once the genes were isolated, they were placed in living animals, such as baby hamsters, which became factories

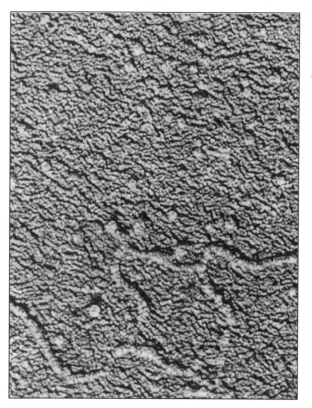

The ability to isolate single DNA strands (two are pictured here) enables doctors to help hemophiliacs.

for producing the clotting proteins, thus bypassing the need for human blood as a source of clotting factors. Since the resulting factor did not involve human blood, there were no viruses and it was considered a safe alternative to factors derived from plasma. This method is known as recombinant DNA technology and was introduced in 1992 as a new treatment for hemophilia. The term *recombinant* simply means the genes are rearranged (recombined) experimentally from a molecule of DNA (the carrier of genetic information inside cells) and placed in a desired order. Before recombinant DNA technology was offered to the general population, it was tested in volunteers for safety. George McCoy, a thirty-nine-year-old hemophiliac, volunteered to be the first patient to receive the new recombinant DNA clotting factor, which did not involve the use of blood. He says, "I felt that genetic engineering and recombinant technology were the best hope for the future because

we knew there was contamination possibility in other products." [17] In the years it took to develop this product, the national
blood supply became safe, but so many in the hemophilia community
had died from AIDS contracted from using human blood that hemophiliacs embraced the new DNA treatment as a safe method
for stopping bleeding without the necessity of using products derived from plasma.

Living and Dying with Hemophilia

While many deaths occurred in the 1980s from AIDS, there were
also many deaths prior to the middle of the twentieth century because of inadequate treatment methods. Before 1970, people with
severe hemophilia often died in childhood or early adulthood
from uncontrollable bleeding episodes. Speaking about what life
was like for a hemophilia one hundred years ago, Kathy Bosma, a
nurse who works with hemophilia patients, says, "Life was so different for people with hemophilia. People weren't expected to live
past 30. Today, we expect people with hemophilia to grow old." [18]
Common causes of death before 1970 were uncontrolled bleeding
after accidents or surgery, or bleeding into vital parts of the body,
like the brain. For those who survived childhood, crippling from
repeated hemorrhages into joints was common. Today, the
lifespan of people with hemophilia, if the AIDS virus has not affected them, is near average. Deaths in the hemophilic population
in the modern era are mostly unrelated to their bleeding disorder.

The history of hemophilia has progressed from a time of little understanding and no effective treatment to great strides in
understanding everything from genetics to how to prevent
bleeds by administering concentrated forms of clotting factors.
These discoveries greatly improve the quality of life for those
with hemophilia.

Chapter 3

Diagnosis and Treatment

H EMOPHILIA IS A disorder in which it is currently possible to know the diagnosis before the first symptoms appear. This was not true in the early twentieth century when the diagnosis of hemophilia depended totally on family history and the symptoms of the patient because diagnostic testing for the disease was not available. Although family history and the patient's symptoms provide enough information to indicate a bleeding disorder, they do not distinguish between hemophilia A and hemophilia B, which require different clotting factors for treatment. Today, tests are available to determine which type of hemophilia the patient has, and to determine if a woman is a carrier of hemophilia. It is also possible to predict with a fair amount of certainty if a pregnant woman's child will develop hemophilia.

Predicting Hemophilia Before Birth

The two tests most often performed to predict the actual disease before birth require obtaining cells from the unborn baby. One test is called chorionic villus sampling (CVS) and is performed by removing a small number of cells from the placenta, which is the thick, pancake-shaped organ inside the mother's uterus through which the baby receives its nourishment during the pregnancy. These cells contain the genetic information of the infant. The test is performed between the second and third months of pregnancy. From this test, the sex of the infant can be determined (important because hemophilia is largely a disease of males), and also knowledge of whether the baby carries the gene for hemophilia.

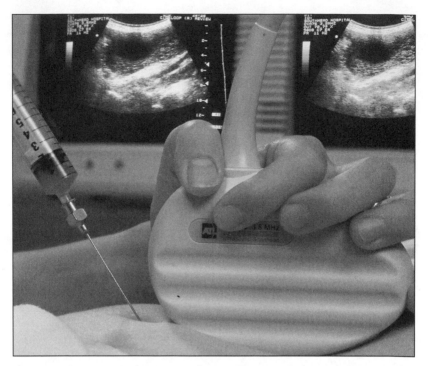

A pregnant woman undergoes amniocentesis, a test that can detect hemophilia.

The second test is called amniocentesis and is performed about four months into a pregnancy. In this test, a long needle is inserted through the abdomen of the mother into her uterus after she has been given medication to numb the area. A small sample of the amniotic fluid surrounding the infant is withdrawn with a syringe. The fluid contains cells with genetic material from the infant's body. This test gives the same information about the infant's chances of having hemophilia that are obtained with chorionic villus sampling, but it cannot be performed as early in the pregnancy. Occasionally, the doctor will want to look at a blood sample from another family member with hemophilia for comparison to aid in reaching a diagnosis.

Blood tests are valuable diagnostic tools because they are used to identify whether a woman carries the hemophilia gene and also to determine which type of hemophilia a child has and how severe it is. In determining carrier status of a woman, two types of tests evaluate the blood for levels of factor VIII and factor IX and the hemophilia gene in the DNA. It takes about two weeks to get results from the DNA test, and it predicts carrier status with 95 to 99 percent accuracy. Testing can sometimes reveal a gene mutation in the mother. Genetic counselor Sarah Cox of the University of Arizona emphasizes the limits of accuracy of the test. "We can't tell families with 100 percent certainty if they're carriers; first we have to identify the mutation, and that's not possible in each case." [19]

Diagnosing Hemophilia After Birth

Once a child is born, tests called factor assays or blood-clotting factor tests can be done to determine hemophilia and its severity. They require withdrawing about two teaspoons of blood from the vein of the child. Specifically, the laboratory performing the test is looking for the percentage of activity of either clotting factor VIII for hemophilia A, or factor IX, also called Christmas factor, for hemophilia B. The lower the percentage of available clotting factor, the more severe the hemophilia is. Levels of factor VIII or IX below 1 percent always represent the most severe form of hemophilia. It takes one to two weeks for the test results to come back.

When making an initial diagnosis of hemophilia, many blood tests besides measuring clotting factors are performed. Since a person's blood might not clot for several reasons besides hemophilia, tests are ordered to rule out bleeding disorders not classified as hemophilia. If the child has hemophilia, these tests will be normal, since the only abnormalities in blood clotting with hemophilia are deficiencies of factors VIII or IX.

Treating Hemophilia

Once testing is completed and the child is diagnosed with hemophilia, treatment begins based on the type of hemophilia found. Treatment is aimed at eliminating symptoms, not curing the disease, since at present there is no cure for hemophilia.

The most common way to treat hemorrhages in hemophiliacs in the United States in the past was to administer the missing factor immediately following the bleed with a concentrated form of the factor. The two forms of clotting factors most often given are freeze-dried factor concentrates derived from human plasma or factors manufactured by recombinant (recombining the order of genes) DNA technology, also freeze-dried. Two criteria are used to decide the dose of factor replacement: the severity of the hemophilia and the weight of the patient. Once dose is determined, sterile water is added to either freeze-dried concentrate (plasma derived or recombinant DNA). The powdered substances come in a container about the size of a salt shaker and are mixed by swirling the bottle, not shaking it, which causes bubbles to form. They are then administered intravenously, meaning a needle is placed in the vein of the patient with tubing connecting the syringe containing the medication to the needle. It takes about twenty to thirty minutes for the medication to infuse. Gerald (J.J.), a nine-year-old with hemophilia A, talks about receiving factor after he bleeds: "Lucky for me that my mom keeps some special medicine in the refrigerator. It's made of this factor VIII. It comes in two vials—one liquid and one powder—and when I need it, she mixes the two together and puts them in a syringe. Then she starts an IV, usually in my hand because I don't like it in my arm. In about five minutes the medicine starts to work."[20] There is one problem with treatment given following a bleed; every bleed, particularly those in joints, has the potential for permanent damage, even if treated promptly.

Treating Bleeds Before They Happen

Prebleed treatment, which was first used in Europe, is gaining popularity in the United States. It is used most frequently with those who have severe hemophilia. With this method, called prophylaxis, meaning prevention, the factor replacement is given on a schedule to prevent bleeds, in contrast to treatment on demand, which waits for a bleed to occur before giving the factors. The main advantage of giving treatment on a prescribed schedule is that it keeps the level of clotting factors high enough to prevent spontaneous bleeds from occurring. This is important because the number one complication of hemophilia bleeds is permanent

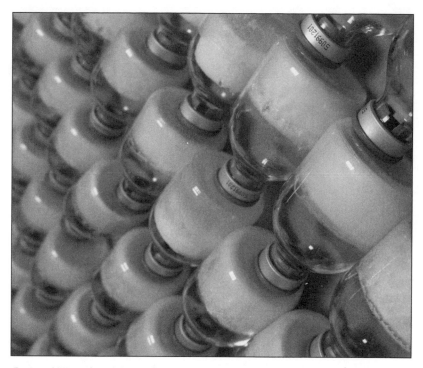

Factors VIII and IX (pictured) are substances derived from human plasma or recombinant DNA to clot blood.

damage to joints, and prebleed treatment nearly eliminates this problem. It is easier to prevent joint damage than it is to treat it once it happens. A typical schedule of infusions is three times a week, but it might be more or less depending on the severity of the condition. Infusions are given in the morning, so the level of factors in the blood stays high during the day's activities. Jay, a seventeen-year-old with severe hemophilia, gave this answer showing how prophylaxis helps him lead an active life: "I play basketball and other sports. Prophylaxis is huge in my being able to play."[21]

The parents of Creighton Peterson, age two, decided on this prebleed treatment after multiple trips to the emergency room starting when he was one and a half years old. After making nine trips over a three-month period to have their child treated for bleeding episodes, Creighton's mother, Ann, said, "We decided to

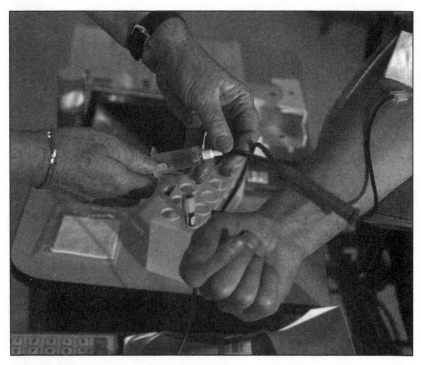

A hemophiliac receives a regular dose of factor replacement to prevent severe bleeding.

take control of our little boy's life."[22] They did this by learning to give the infusions to him on a schedule at home, so he would not experience unexpected bleeds.

The disadvantages to prophylaxis (prebleed treatment) center on three issues: the greater number of infusions required, the high cost of the factor, and the need to locate a vein for each infusion. Usually, when a family decides on prebleed treatment, an upper chest vein is located on the child by minor surgical procedure, and a port is implanted under the skin with the blood vessel encased in it. This port can be used over and over and allows immediate entry into the vein without the necessity of searching for a new vein with each infusion. An alternate method to prevent multiple needle sticks is an external catheter threaded into a vein, which can stay in place for months at a time with proper care. External catheters are a type of IV inserted by a professional into the bend of the elbow (medically referred to as the antecubital fossa) and threaded up the arm so the tip of the catheter lies in a larger blood vessel than is available in the hand or lower arm, where most IVs are inserted. Both implanted IV ports and external catheters add to the cost of treatment.

The Expense of Treatment

Hemophilia is one of the most expensive diseases to treat. The average annual cost of treatment for a hemophiliac is between $50,000 and $200,000. Since amount of clotting factor is based on weight, it costs more for an adult to be treated than a child. The Great Lakes Hemophilia Foundation gave the following cost estimates per infusion for four age groups. The cost for one treatment for a baby is over $100, for a five-year-old over $300, for an adolescent over $600, and for an adult male over $1,000. Because prebleed treatments are given several times a week, the cost of administering the factors is higher than the cost for treating only when a bleed occurs. Treatment costs are so expensive because of all the research and technology that has gone into developing the newer products. The positive side is that this same technology has decreased complications and made treatment safer.

Other Treatments Used

For cases of mild hemophilia A, a drug called DDAVP (desmopressin) is sometimes used for treatment instead of clotting factors. The medication was developed in 1977, but not licensed for use in the United States until 1984. It is classified as a hormone, which is a chemical normally produced by the body whose function is to regulate the activity of another part of the body. DDAVP is a medication that works like a natural hormone called antidiuretic hormone (ADH), normally secreted by the pituitary gland in the brain. It is ordered by the physician according to the weight of the person and works by increasing the blood concentration of factor VIII. An additional way it is thought to help is by assisting platelets to adhere to the site of injury in the blood vessel. DDAVP is administered into a vein like clotting factors or is available as a nasal spray.

DDAVP is advantageous to use because it is not derived from human blood, so it carries no risk of HIV contamination because it is a hormone and not a blood product. Cost is another factor in its favor, since an average dose of DDAVP costs $100, as compared with between $400 and $1,000 for a dose of factor VIII. The disadvantage is its limited use, since only those with mild hemophilia A benefit from it.

Physical therapy is another important treatment for hemophilia. Physical therapists use stretching, movement exercises, and weight lifting with hemophilia patients. Other treatments employed may include splints, ice, heat, ultrasound, nerve stimulation, and water therapy, which creates less stress on joints than weight-bearing exercises while providing necessary exercise.

One way physical therapy exercises help hemophiliacs is to decrease bleeds by strengthening the muscles around the joints

Hemophiliacs often undergo physical therapy to strengthen muscles around joints most susceptible to bleeding.

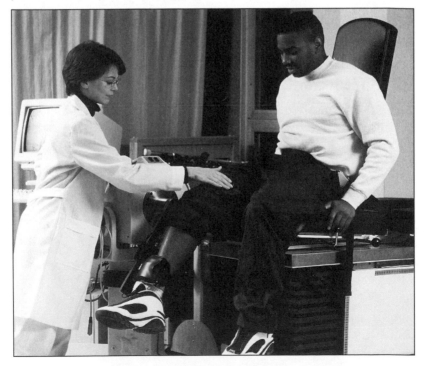

most likely to bleed in a person. Steve Houghton, a physical therapist at Michigan State University's Bleeding Disorders Clinic, says,

> When factor product wasn't readily available in the 1970s, inactivity was the rule, but the joints just got worse and worse. It was a vicious cycle—if a joint bleeds, it causes pain and is used less, so it becomes weaker and more prone to re-bleeding. That's why physical therapy is so important. It helps maintain the range of motion and strength. If you look at patients with arthritis, who have musculoskeletal problems similar to people with hemophilia, the principles of strengthening and stretching are used with great success. When we started to prescribe this for hemophilia patients, bleeds decreased and so did areas of disability in the joints.[23]

The second way physical therapy is used is to help patients regain range of motion and increase strength following bleeding into a joint. Initially, the joint is moved gently to prevent stiffness after bleeding ceases. Following recovery from the bleeding, strengthening exercises are added to decrease chances of permanent joint damage. A complete program of rehabilitation can last six to nine months.

Medications to Avoid

Hemophiliacs must constantly be aware of products capable of making their condition worse. The majority of these affect the body's ability to clot blood. Two medications avoided are aspirin and a group of drugs referred to as NSAIDs (nonsteroidal anti-inflammatory drugs). Aspirin and NSAIDs are commonly given for pain and inflammation in arthritis, but they are contraindicated (not advised) for similar problems in hemophiliacs. Both of these drugs interfere with the clumping of platelets, one of the steps necessary for blood to clot. Vitamin E also prolongs blood clotting and is avoided. Because all medications have side effects, hemophiliacs consult doctors before taking any medication not prescribed.

First Aid for Minor Bleeds

Knowledge of first aid is important for anyone having contact with a hemophiliac. Not all bleeds require replacement of clotting factors; most external bleeds are controlled by the same methods used to stop bleeding in anyone. The first step is to apply pressure to the bleeding area to close the blood vessel. In using this method for the hemophiliac, pressure is applied for five to ten minutes, which is longer than for a person with normal clotting. A second measure to employ is ice or an ice pack, wrapped in cloth and applied to the site, which constricts the blood vessel and slows bleeding. An alternate way to apply cold is to use a towel dipped in ice water. Cold is left on the wound for no longer than fifteen or twenty minutes per application, since longer times can cause tissue damage. If possible, elevating the body part above the level of the heart also slows bleeding, as does limiting movement until the bleeding stops. Once bleeding is controlled, the area is bandaged.

The Physician Specialist and Hemophilia Treatment Centers

Today, hemophiliacs have more control over their illness and treatment than before; however, a physician specialist needs to manage the illness and be available for problems. The doctor most qualified to care for a hemophilia patient is a hematologist, a doctor who specializes in diseases of the blood and the immune system. A hematologist is a physician who has graduated from medical school, has completed several additional years of study in the field of internal medicine, and then has specialized further in blood and immune system disorders. These physicians receive certification in their specialty by passing an exam in hematology.

Many hematologists work at hemophilia treatment centers. The purpose of a hemophilia treatment center (HTC) is to offer complete up-to-date care by professionals educated about hemophilia. HTCs were established in the United States in 1975 and receive federal money to help with operating costs. There are approximately 130 centers, which employ hematologists, nurses, social workers, dentists, and physical therapists. Tina Bullard of North Carolina says about the hemophilia center her family uses,

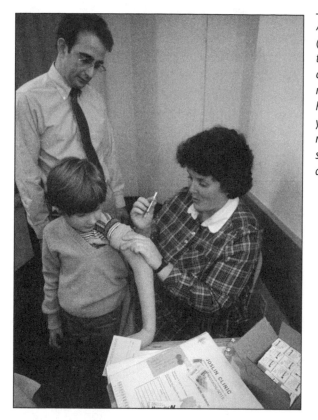

At an HTC (hemophilia treatment center), a young patient receives care from a hematologist; young hemophiliacs miss less school by seeking treatment at HTCs.

"The Comprehensive Hemophilia Center at Chapel Hill is staffed by the most caring individuals I have ever met. It has been a very positive experience to know them, and the first experience could not have been warmer."[24] The National Hemophilia Foundation has a list of hemophilia treatment centers, so patients can locate one close to their homes.

The benefits of using an HTC are many. Studies have shown that patients receiving treatment at a hemophilia treatment center lose less time at school and on the job because of their illness. The death rate for hemophiliacs treated at hemophilia centers is 40 percent lower than for those treated elsewhere. This lower death rate is attributed to care by professionals who have experience with hemophilia on a daily basis and are knowledgeable about the latest treatments. Services at HTCs include everything from diagnosis to dental care and patient education.

Hemophilia treatment centers promote the use of home-infusion programs so that bleeding episodes are treated immediately. Hemophilia centers teach parents of young children, and boys approaching their teen years, to give their own infusions at home. This is important because the longer the wait for treatment, such as often occurs in emergency rooms, the greater the chance of a serious complication. Zack Dansker recalls the decision to stick himself with a needle the first time: "I'd wanted to self-infuse for a long time, but I was afraid." [25] Zack learned how to self-infuse just after he turned eleven, while attending a summer camp for hemophiliacs. His instructor was "Dr." Bob, a physician's assistant from one of the local hemophilia treatment centers.

Ethical Dilemmas

In addition to making the decision to learn self-infusion, families of hemophiliacs are often faced with choosing between a blood supply that has not always been safe or no treatment altogether. Donors and donated blood have been tested since 1986, which has eliminated some of the problems of the transmission of the diseases AIDS and hepatitis; still, hemophiliacs are concerned that the newer nonplasma recombinant DNA factors may have side effects not yet recognized. The hemophilia population is understandably wary of the safety of treatments after the number of deaths that occurred in the 1980s from freeze-dried clotting factor manufactured from human plasma contaminated with HIV. One of the concerns about HIV transmission is that it can be present in a donor's blood, but antibodies will not show up on a conventional blood test for as long as six months after infection with the virus. The Food and Drug Administration in early 2002 approved a new blood screening test for detection of HIV and hepatitis C virus that can detect the presence of these deadly viruses in a donor's blood only days after infection rather than months. This is a significant discovery further reducing the chances that a hemophiliac will be exposed to AIDS or hepatitis C through blood products.

Another problem for hemophiliacs is the occasional shortage of clotting factors and who gets them. This shortage applies to both plasma-derived clotting factors and nonplasma DNA clotting factors. Clotting factors from human plasma depend on the number of blood donations, which vary over time, since most donations occur voluntarily. Manufactured clotting factors can also undergo shortages because of contaminants in the product or other manufacturing problems. When a shortage occurs, the prescribing physician is faced with decisions about who needs the product most and who needs which type of clotting factor—plasma-derived or recombinant DNA. Some hemophiliacs are reluctant to change brands or use alternate sources of clotting factors. This means the physician must make a difficult decision about which patient receives the available supply.

From initial diagnosis to choosing a treatment method, the family of a hemophiliac and the patient stay informed and involved. The diagnosis of hemophilia is frightening, and families of children with hemophilia are immediately faced with many decisions about care. Whether the patient chooses home infusion or emergency room care by professionals depends on the severity of the disease and the willingness of the family to learn infusion techniques. Fortunately, the twenty-first century offers more and better options than at any time in the past.

Chapter 4

Complications

A LTHOUGH CURRENT TREATMENT for hemophilia has lessened complications, they still occur. The three most important complications affecting those with hemophilia A and B are: (1) damage to joints from repeated bleeds, (2) the development of inhibitors, a response by the body's immune system making treatment ineffective, and (3) infection with viruses carried in blood, such as hepatitis and HIV (human immunodeficiency virus). In addition, brain hemorrhage, while not a common complication, can be extremely serious.

Joint Deformities

Joint deformities are the number one complication of uncontrolled bleeding. The joints most often damaged are knees, ankles, and elbows, with hip and shoulder joints bleeding less often. Hemophiliacs frequently have one joint, known as a "target" joint, which bleeds more often than others. Ryan White, a young hemophiliac, described joint bleeding in this way: "A bleed occurs from a broken blood vessel or vein. The blood then had nowhere to go so it would swell up in a joint. You could compare it to trying to pour a quart of milk into a pint-sized container of milk." [26]

Even one serious joint bleed, medically called hemarthrosis, can begin the process of permanent damage. More commonly, the damage results from many bleeds into the same joint. The damage to a joint that a hemophiliac receives is very similar to the damage in an arthritic joint. Severe adult hemophiliacs, who grew up before prophylactic (prebleed) treatment was common, almost always have some joint deformity. Younger hemophiliacs who receive prophylactic treatment often escape deformities.

One of the problems with joint bleeding is its tendency to become worse with each episode of bleeding. One part of the joint damaged is the inside joint lining, called the synovium, which lubricates the joint. The synovium has a large number of blood vessels, causing it to bleed easily. With each bleed, the synovium becomes thicker and grows more blood vessels, making each subsequent bleed more severe.

The pain that accompanies a bleed into a joint is severe. Because of the rigid structure of the bony area, the blood is trapped in the joint, causing it to swell until, over a period of time, the synovium can reabsorb the blood. A man named Adam H., who remembers his boyhood with hemophilia in the 1940s, says, "You wouldn't bleed to death from a bad knee—but the pain would be rather unpleasant. When it got really bad, you'd call one of the doctors. He'd come out at midnight and give me a shot of morphine. On a

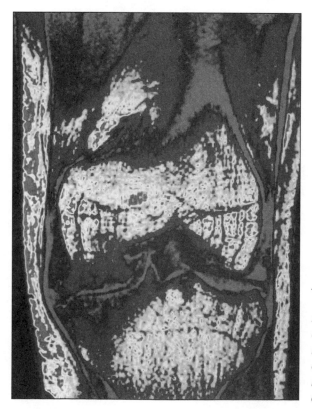

This MRI scan shows osteoarthritis of the knee joint, a condition similar to hemophilic arthropathy.

few occasions when even that didn't work, my rabbi would come over and almost literally spend the night with me. I guess in many respects, it wasn't a very pleasant childhood."[27]

While severe pain is mostly temporary, the damage to joints, known as hemophilic arthropathy, is not. The prefix *arthro-* means "joint" and the suffix *-pathy* means "disease," so *arthropathy* means "disease of the joints." Depending on the joint involved, arthropathy affects the ability to kneel, write without pain, ride a bicycle, or dance, and might even mean the necessity of using a wheelchair or crutches. Treatment for joint arthropathy is physical therapy as prescribed by a physician or therapist. At the time of the actual bleed, ice packs, splinting, and avoidance of weight-bearing exercise are the usual treatments in addition to the administration of clotting factors.

The Body Fights the Treatment

Although joint deformities are becoming a thing of the past, the development of inhibitors (antibodies to the clotting factor) still occurs. Every person, whether or not they have hemophilia, manufactures antibodies, which act like an army to protect the body against foreign invaders. Most of the time this is beneficial. The development of inhibitors/antibodies by the person with hemophilia, however, interferes with needed treatment. The inhibitors attack infused clotting factors as something foreign and destroy the factors before they can stop the bleeding.

No one knows for sure why some hemophiliacs develop inhibitors and others do not. Inhibitors affect between 14 and 25 percent of those with severe hemophilia A, but only about 2 to 3 percent of those with hemophilia B. Inhibitors develop in hemophiliacs in approximately the same percentages regardless of whether the person is treated with plasma-derived clotting factors or recombinant DNA clotting factors.

Detection of inhibitors occurs in one of two ways. One way uses blood tests to detect inhibitors (antibodies). A second method relies on the observation powers of the patient and family. With this method, the patient or family notices that clotting factors that formerly controlled bleeding no longer work. This is an indication that inhibitors are attacking the clotting factors, rendering them ineffective.

Treatment for the unwanted production of inhibitors is called immune tolerance therapy (ITT). Immune tolerance therapy works much better with hemophilia A than hemophilia B because many with hemophilia B have an allergic reaction to the treatment. The purpose is to get the body's immune system used to the clotting factors needed to prevent bleeding, so eventually the production of inhibitors ceases. The method has some similarities to desensitization treatments (allergy shots) given to people with allergies. With desensitization shots for allergies, the patient is administered the very thing that he is allergic to in increasing doses so his body will become accustomed to it. In immune tolerance therapy, the hemophiliac also receives the substance his body is reacting against—in this case, the clotting factors necessary to stop bleeding. The difference between allergy shots and immune tolerance therapy is that clotting factors are not gradually introduced to the hemophiliac, but are given in very large doses. A hematologist closely monitors the high doses of the clotting factor, which are given on a daily, or sometimes twice-daily, basis in order to get the body accustomed to the factor. This procedure can take from one to twenty-four months and costs more than $1 million a year.

An alternate way to treat inhibitors is to change the product used to stop bleeding. Use of recombinant factor VIII has helped some patients with inhibitors. Debbie Best of California says, "[My son] Billy Joe had an inhibitor from the time he was 3 years old to 7 years old. Only the factor product was changed [as a way to treat it], and we needed an extra lab test every other month. I guess we took it as a normal thing that happens to people with hemophilia."[28]

Drugs to suppress the body's immune system, which manufactures inhibitors, are sometimes tried as less expensive alternatives before attempting immune tolerance therapy. The success rate for suppressing inhibitors by all methods is 60 to 80 percent.

Though human body organs produce beneficial antibodies, these can interfere with hemophiliacs' clotting treatments.

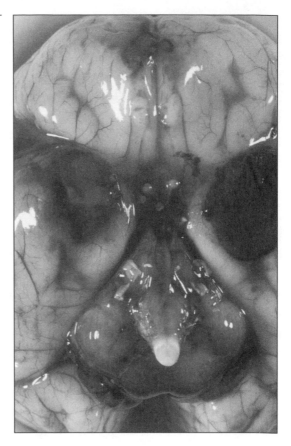

A Potentially Deadly Bleed

While not as common a complication as joint deformities or the development of inhibitors, any head injury in a person with hemophilia is considered life threatening. Intracranial hemorrhage (bleeding into the brain) is the leading cause of death for hemophiliacs other than death from AIDS. A buildup of blood in the brain can result in permanent brain damage as well as death. The brain has a high concentration of the clotting factor thromboplastin, so hemorrhages here occur less frequently than other areas; nevertheless, even a suspected head injury is reason enough to seek medical attention. Bleeding in the head is considered when there is a history of any minor head injury or the person has a severe unexplained headache lasting more than four hours.

Dr. Peter S. Smith, director of a hospital pediatric hematology department, gives an example of a head injury that was treated in time. He described a minor head injury in a young boy whose only symptom was a headache. His parents took the initiative to administer clotting factors to their son because they knew he hit his head. Dr. Smith says, "The symptoms were in fact from an intracranial bleed, but because it was treated so quickly, the child has had no resulting neurological problems. What was important was the rapidity with which everything was done." [29]

Later, more serious, symptoms of intracranial bleeding are nausea and vomiting, listlessness, difficulty staying awake, double vision, slurred speech, or weakness in the arms or legs. In the case of head injuries in a hemophiliac, the bleeding may or may not be visible to an observer, but is treated with factor replacement immediately on the presumption that bleeding is occurring. Physicians usually do not wait for CAT (computerized axial tomography) scans or other diagnostic tests before treating because of the potential seriousness of bleeding into the brain tissue.

Infected Blood and the Liver

A more common complication of hemophilia than brain hemorrhage is hepatitis, which is transmitted by infected blood. Viruses cause hepatitis, which affects the liver by causing inflammation. Since the liver manufactures many of the body's clotting factors, hepatitis is a special danger to hemophiliacs who may experience a further decrease in their body's ability to clot blood, in addition to other damage done to the liver by the disease. Hepatitis is transmitted in several ways, but most hemophiliacs infected with hepatitis are infected through exposure to blood or blood products containing the virus. A total of six types of hepatitis have been identified—hepatitis A, B, C, D, E, and G. Hemophiliacs are at risk for types A, B, and C.

In the general population, hepatitis A is transmitted by the intake of food or water contaminated with the virus. The virus is found in the stool of an infected person, so hand washing after using the bathroom and before eating is the most effective way to prevent spread of the virus. Infected hemophiliacs have contracted hepatitis A through treatment with clotting factors extracted from human plasma. No one knows how this occurred, since this is not the usual route of transmission of hepatitis A. Symptoms of hepatitis A are fever, nausea, jaundice (yellowing of the skin), and tiredness. The disease usually runs its course in about two months. A two-injection vaccine exists for hepatitis A and is available to anyone two years of age or older. The vaccine is highly recommended for people with hemophilia.

Hepatitis B also affects the liver, but is a more serious illness than hepatitis A, since some people who are infected never fully recover, and some even die from it. Studies indicate that hepatitis B virus is one hundred times more likely to infect a person than the virus causing AIDS. Hepatitis B is spread by blood or blood products contaminated with the virus. This puts hemophiliacs at greater risk than most people, since one treatment choice is receiving blood-derived products.

Symptoms for hepatitis B are very similar to symptoms for hepatitis A and include nausea, fever, jaundice, and extreme tiredness. Thirty to 40 percent of people who have hepatitis B have no symptoms and can unintentionally pass the virus to other people. While all blood is now tested for blood-borne diseases, many hemophiliacs were infected with hepatitis B before 1987. The Centers for Disease Control recommend that all hemophiliacs, as well as all children, be vaccinated against hepatitis B by receiving a series of three shots to protect against the virus.

The third type of hepatitis is known as hepatitis C and is the major cause of chronic liver disease; in rare cases it can progress to liver cancer if not treated. Liver failure with the need for a liver transplant is also a possibility. Half of the nearly four thousand liver transplants performed in 1995 in the United States were for chronic cases of hepatitis C. Kathleen Cadmus, a registered nurse, testified before the Ohio Senate Health Committee in 1997, and said, "In a study done with our hemophilia patients at the Ohio State University [OSU] in 1996, 87 percent of persons from 27 Ohio counties receiving care for their bleeding disorder at OSU were hepatitis C positive [meaning they were infected with hepatitis C]." [30]

Hepatitis C is spread mainly by contact with blood or blood products, but can also be spread by sharing needles, razors, toothbrushes, or earrings. Hepatitis C is dangerous because often the person infected has no symptoms, but the disease is still damaging to the liver and can be transmitted to others. If the person has symptoms, they are similar to those for hepatitis A and B. There is currently no vaccine against hepatitis C, although treatment with antiviral drugs is available. Since 1991, no cases of hepatitis C contracted through blood transfusions or blood products have occurred in the United States, because blood donors are screened for hepatitis C and blood products are treated to kill viruses. Before this time, hepatitis C was the most common form of hepatitis acquired from blood transfusions and blood products.

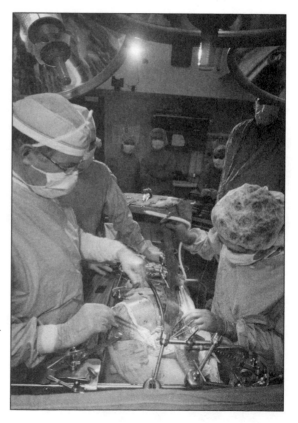

Liver transplants are sometimes performed on hemophiliacs if chronic hepatitis leads to liver failure.

The AIDS Epidemic

Hepatitis is not the only disease hemophiliacs were exposed to through use of blood products. In the early to middle 1980s, many hemophiliacs received blood products contaminated with HIV (human immunodeficiency virus). The human immunodeficiency virus, unknown prior to the early 1980s, is incurable once a person is infected. HIV progresses through four disease stages to the final one, AIDS (acquired immunodeficiency syndrome). As the name suggests, the virus attacks a person's immune system, increasing susceptibility to illnesses like pneumonia, fungal infections, and some cancers. One of the methods of transmission is through contact with blood. In the 1980s, the factor products given to hemophiliacs came from human plasma, the liquid portion of blood. Individual blood donations lacked enough clotting factor, so the products were made from pools of donors—sometimes 15,000 to 60,000 people. Therefore, the chances of the product containing HIV were enormous. Until 1985, mandatory screening of blood donors for HIV was not required. As a result, in the 1980s, half of all hemophiliacs became infected with HIV through contaminated factor products, and 90 percent of those with severe hemophilia were infected because of their greater use of blood products. In 2002, the Centers for Disease Control estimated there were 5,000 AIDS cases in adults and adolescents with hemophilia, and 237 hemophilic children under thirteen had AIDS. Ryan White, a hemophiliac, discovered he had AIDS at age thirteen following a hospital admission for surgery. He said, "I came face to face with death at thirteen years old. I was diagnosed with AIDS: a killer." [31]

Ryan White, Hemophilia, and AIDS

Ryan White was diagnosed with severe hemophilia at the age of three days. Since he was born in 1971, the newer treatments of cryoprecipitate and freeze-dried clotting factors from human plasma were available to help with his bleeding problems. This should have ensured a fairly normal lifestyle for him, but this was before blood donors and blood products were tested for HIV. In 1984, just after his

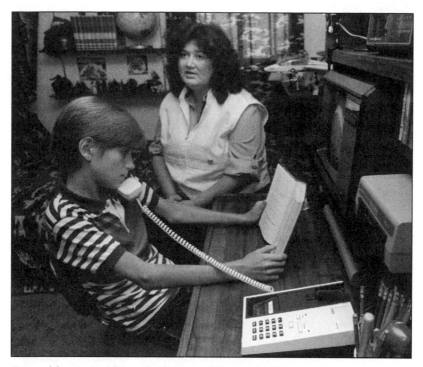

Banned from attending school, hemophiliac and AIDS patient Ryan White telecommutes to his classes before his death at age eighteen.

thirteenth birthday, he learned from a physician that he had contracted AIDS from contaminated clotting factors.

In the 1980s, people were just learning about HIV and AIDS, and many were fearful that the virus could infect them through casual contact. The school Ryan attended refused to let him continue classes, and people avoided him and his family. Ryan and his family sued the school district to allow him to attend classes, but although they won the case, he was treated so badly by the students that the family finally moved to another town. In the new town, the students had been educated about the AIDS virus, and his experience was much better. Because of his problems and the publicity he received, Ryan became a celebrity, appearing on talk shows educating people about AIDS and participating in charity events with famous people. A television movie called *The Ryan White Story* was made about his life when he was sixteen.

In April 1990, at the age of eighteen, Ryan White died of AIDS. He had lived five and a half years from the time of his AIDS diagnosis. Four months after his death, Congress passed the Ryan White Care Act, designed to help states, communities, and families cope with AIDS by providing needed money for AIDS clinics and uninsured individuals. The Ryan White Care Act also educates health care professionals in the treatment of HIV and provides dental care for AIDS victims.

Ricky Ray Hemophilia Relief Fund

The story of Ricky Ray has many similarities to the story of Ryan White. Ricky Ray was the oldest of three brothers with hemophilia. He and his two younger brothers, Robert and Randy, not only had hemophilia but also were diagnosed with HIV from tainted blood clotting factors. Like Ryan White, they were barred from attending public school after the diagnosis of HIV and had to obtain a court order allowing them back in school. They were so persecuted for having the virus that their Florida home was burned to the ground by arsonists. Both Ricky and his brother Robert progressed from being HIV positive (meaning their blood contained the human immunodeficiency virus) to having full-blown AIDS. Although Ricky was young, he became an activist for AIDS by writing letters to U.S. presidents in the 1980s and early 1990s, asking them to increase AIDS funding. In 1992, at the age of fifteen, Ricky Ray died from AIDS; a few years later, his brother Robert, who lived to age twenty-two, also died of AIDS. Calvin Dawson of Florida, whose hemophiliac brother, Marvin Dawson, died of AIDS in the early 1990s, made this comment: "There are a lot of angry, bitter people out there. They feel that it didn't need to happen to Ricky Ray, and it doesn't have to happen to them."[32]

As a result of Ricky Ray's efforts, others were inspired to take up the cause of hemophiliacs infected with HIV. Because they continued fighting for Ricky Ray's beliefs, Congress passed the Ricky Ray Hemophilia Relief Fund Act in 1998 to compensate victims of hemophilia who were infected with HIV from blood products. This act acknowledged that blood contaminated with dangerous viruses had been sold to hemophiliacs and others with blood coagulation disorders, who were not warned of the dangers even though evidence existed as early as 1982 that the products could be contaminated. The government was therefore held accountable for failing to regulate the plasma industry.

The Ricky Ray Act compensated hemophiliac/HIV patients with $100,000 each as a compassionate gesture for the harm experienced. This was a small amount, considering that the annual cost of care for a patient diagnosed with both hemophilia and HIV is $160,000 and HIV can lead to full-blown AIDS, which is terminal. Peggy Hesselbacher, the mother of a hemophilia patient with AIDS, says, "It still isn't enough. What amount of money can possibly make up for a life?"[33]

Of the five complications, only the problem of inhibitors continues to plague new hemophiliacs. At present, there is no way to

Hemophiliacs are at risk for contracting HIV and hepatitis from contaminated blood. These lab workers test donated blood for such maladies.

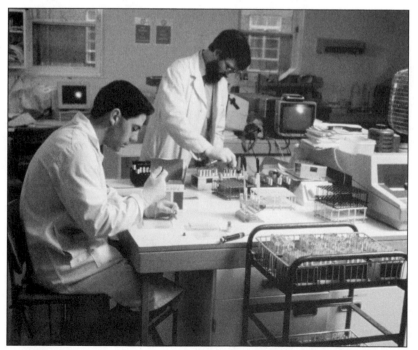

prevent the formation of inhibitors; there is only treatment once the problem is known. Joint deformities remain a problem for older severe hemophiliacs who received on-demand treatment, but are rarely a problem for younger hemophiliacs, who receive prebleed treatment, which prevents most joint damage. Intracranial bleeding can still occur, but knowledgeable families of hemophiliacs now know to take all head injuries seriously and, when in doubt, treat. The best news is that treating blood and blood products and screening donors for harmful viruses have virtually eliminated the worry that hepatitis and HIV will be transmitted through blood sources. There have been no known cases of hepatitis A and B or HIV from blood clotting products since 1986, and no known cases of hepatitis C being contracted from factors since 1991. This means that hemophilia today is a disease that can be managed with minimal complications.

Chapter 5

Living with Hemophilia—An Accident Waiting to Happen

DESPITE THE NORMALITY of life for most hemophiliacs in the twenty-first century, hemophiliacs still face many challenges and decisions throughout their lives. Decisions can range from a child deciding on a sport to participate in, to a young adult with a family history of hemophilia considering its impact on a decision to have children. The challenge of hemophilia is one for the entire family, not just the patient, since all family members are affected by living with a person with a chronic illness. However, wise choices, made from sound information, give the best chance for a normal life for the patient as well as the family.

Sports

One of the decisions that hemophiliacs face is what sports are safe, given the severity of their hemophilia. Those with mild hemophilia have more choices than those with severe hemophilia. The majority of hemophiliacs are aware that participation in sports is beneficial as long as sensible choices are made, because regular exercise keeps joints strong by providing muscular support. Swimming is the number one sport universally agreed by physicians as safe for hemophiliacs. Swimming protects joints by developing muscles around them, but does not put undue strain on them. The risk of being bumped or jostled is low compared with other sports. Golf is also a sport most physicians agree is safe for even severe hemophiliacs. Perry Parker is a hemophiliac who plays golf professionally. He also works with young boys with hemophilia to teach them how to safely participate in sports by demonstrating proper techniques. Perry has a brother, Corey, also a hemophiliac, who is a professional baseball player.

According to the Canadian Hemophilia Society, other sports that put low stress on joints are bicycling, tennis, and running. Paul McNeil is a registered nurse in Canada who has hemophilia B (Christmas disease). With careful training, he was able to run the Canadian International Marathon in 2000, but agrees that the stress of a marathon would not be suitable for all hemophiliacs. Weight lifting, using light to medium handheld weights, can be helpful in building muscles as long as proper technique is em-

Because swimming is a low-impact sport it is an often recommended activity for hemophiliacs.

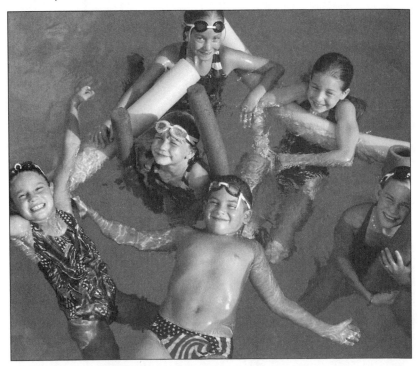

ployed. Weight lifting with heavy weights is not recommended because of the danger of injuring muscles that provide the support for joints.

Those with mild hemophilia may be able to play soccer or baseball, or even ski. Skateboarding, rollerblading, and horseback riding, however, are all considered high-risk sports because the risk of falling with resultant serious injury is higher than for other activities. Hemophiliacs are warned not to participate in sports when their joints are swollen and painful.

Certain physical activities are considered off-limits for all with hemophilia. These activities are mostly contact sports like football, wrestling, boxing, and ice hockey. Participation in contact sports puts a high degree of stress on joints and can lead to bleeding episodes.

Depending on the sport, protective gear may be needed for athletic hemophiliacs. Fortunately, today most children wear helmets, pads, or gloves when biking or batting at baseball, so this is not considered unusual. It is not necessary to wear protective gear for activities that normally do not require it. Many medical professionals believe that this practice puts too much focus on the illness and is counterproductive.

Developmental Issues

Another area that impacts children with hemophilia is developmental milestones and how those affect a child with hemophilia. Each new age level brings different issues regarding the illness.

How children cope with hemophilia is largely determined by age. Preschoolers, who have limited understanding, often cry or fight back during treatments requiring a needle. To cope with such treatment, which preschoolers sometimes see as a form of punishment, they often revert to comforting behavior like thumb sucking.

Full understanding of why treatment is necessary usually does not happen until age six or seven. School-aged children are old enough and knowledgeable enough to recognize and report signs of internal bleeding.

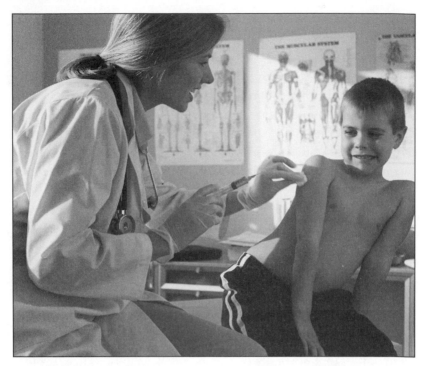

Young children living with hemophilia may experience apprehension in treating their disease.

Adolescence is a difficult time for a hemophiliac because teenagers want to fit in, not stand out as different. Some teen hemophiliacs deliberately engage in risky behavior in an attempt to deny the seriousness of their disorder. Audrey Taylor, a hemophilia nurse coordinator, says, "One of the biggest concerns with this age group is letting bleeds get out of hand because they don't want to rest or miss activities."[34] In addition, emotional feelings concerning hemophilia can peak during this age.

The limitations put on lifestyle by hemophilia can damage self-esteem, which is the amount of worth people attribute to themselves. Children learn self-esteem early in life through success in everyday activities and through treatment by other people. Hemophiliacs recognize early that their life is different from others and may feel afraid, powerless, or angry. Having strong support from family members is important in coping with hemophilia. Allowing children to choose activities they excel at and enjoy helps develop good self-esteem. Failure to adapt to the disease can lead to isolation and a decrease in job and social opportunities.

School Days

Hemophilia is a disease that requires information to be shared with anyone who has contact with the child for an extended time, including day care workers, school nurses, and teachers. Because of the rareness of the disease, even school nurses may have little experience with hemophilia and may need additional education.

Day care and preschool workers receive formal in-service training from an experienced hemophilia nurse. In addition, they must be knowledgeable about first aid for external bleeds. The responsibility of parents is to provide an emergency care plan in case their child has a bleed, and they must let staff know their main responsibility is to notify the parents immediately, especially when there is the possibility of an internal bleed.

Children with hemophilia can be in regular classrooms and participate in regular activities. By the time a child is school aged, he can report symptoms of internal bleeds to his teachers. The type of bleeding hemophiliacs experience always allows for time to call for help. Although the bleeding lasts longer, it is not faster, so calling 9-1-1 is usually not necessary.

Summer Camps

Camps for hemophiliacs are designed to provide a sense of normalcy by planning outdoor fun and a chance to meet other hemophiliac children and their families. Nearly every state has one camp available for hemophiliacs. The National Hemophilia Foundation provides a list of available camps with information about each one.

Most camps last a week, are staffed with professional medical people, and admit campers ages six to nineteen, depending on the camp. Some camps also sponsor educational programs for parents while their children enjoy activities such as talent shows, boating, swimming, hiking, fishing, and crafts. Many camps teach willing children to self-infuse clotting factors for the first time as part of the week's activities.

Costs for a week of camp can range from free to hundreds of dollars. However, many camps receive supplemental funds from state hemophilia organizations, corporations, and individuals and are able to offer very low-cost camping. Actor Paul Newman contributes money for camps for children with serious illnesses. These camps, named Hole in the Wall Gang, are located in Connecticut and Florida.

Careers

One of the big steps in becoming independent is choosing a career. Hemophiliacs have nearly as many job opportunities as others, with only a few exceptions. Those with hemophilia generally are not good candidates for hazardous jobs where injury is a possibility. However, manual labor, for the most part, does not have to be avoided.

According to the National Hemophilia Foundation, those with severe hemophilia have sometimes encountered discrimination by prospective employers, although it is illegal to discriminate because of physical problems as long as a person is capable of performing the job. Val Bias of California says, "I only told my immediate supervisor about my hemophilia after I had the job and usually after I had proven myself in some way. If it wasn't hazardous work, or if my hemophilia wouldn't interfere with my ability to do the work, then I didn't tell. People may disagree with this philosophy, but my career is not about hemophilia, it is about my ability, my competence, and my skill." [35]

Marriage and Having Children

Along with choosing a career, marriage and a family are important. A person with a family history of hemophilia might wish to consult a genetic counselor before having children. A genetic counselor is a medical professional with special training in diseases that are inherited. The counselor's job is to look at the patient's family history to determine the risk of transmitting genetic diseases to future children and then relay this knowledge to the

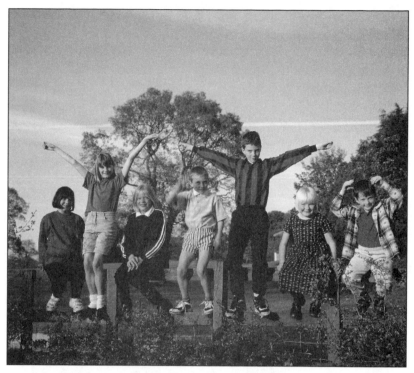

Young hemophiliacs get the chance to meet others like them at an outdoor summer camp.

patient. Once information is received, prospective parents can use it to decide whether they want to have children and risk transmission of the disease.

If the prospective parents choose to have children and one or more of the children has hemophilia, mothers in particular usually feel guilty, since mothers pass the gene to sons by their X chromosome. Rachel Stuart, nurse coordinator at Phoenix Children's Hospital Hemophilia Center, says, "Moms often feel responsible for their son's condition, and I tell them it's not their fault at all. You don't get to pick which genes you pass on—it's a totally random roll of the dice." [36]

The Affect of Hemophilia on the Family

Parents of a child with hemophilia may be overprotective or permissive. Because of the potential consequences of an unchecked

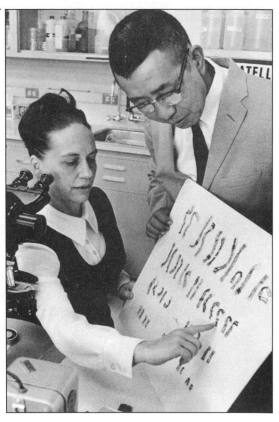

Dr. Margery Shaw and Dr. T.C. Hsu discuss a process of marking genes to identify birth defects and genetic diseases like hemophilia.

bleeding episode, parents often want to shield their child from any situation in which he might be injured. This type of parent sets many limits on the child's activities. An anonymous mother commented in *Raising a Child with Hemophilia*, "My husband became overprotective when our son began to walk. He would hover near him and expect me to hover over him, too. He tried to avoid injuries by carrying our son everywhere. But our son began to resent this. My husband became more upset than I whenever our son got hurt and felt the need to blame one of us."[37]

The opposite situation is a parent who is too permissive. Parents who react this way attempt to make up for the restrictions of hemophilia by letting the child have or do whatever he wants. In other words, there are no rules about acceptable behavior and they are exempt from helping with routine household chores.

Hemophilia affects all family members including siblings. The brother or sister of a hemophiliac may feel neglected because of the amount of attention the affected child receives. Sisters, as they grow older and learn how the disease is transmitted, may worry about the possibility of their being carriers. Experts on hemophilia say it is common for brothers or sisters to sometimes be jealous of or be angry with the child who has hemophilia. Negative feelings are handled by allowing appropriate expression, by teaching brothers or sisters about hemophilia, and by parents setting aside time to spend with the unaffected child. Elaine Guffey of Missouri relates the effect hemophilia had on her son's older brother: "It was hard for Jimmy at first because he is the oldest, has no hemophilia, and was used to getting all the attention. I just show him he is loved and is as important to me as Brandon, in his own special way. I show that his feelings count. I talk to him at length if anything is upsetting him." [38]

Choosing Where to Live

The decision about where to live is another issue that can cause stress for the family of a hemophiliac. Living in an area distant from a hemophilia treatment center means that a nonspecialist in hemophilia may be the only choice for care. Although there are more than 130 hemophilia treatment centers in the United States, some hemophiliacs live in rural areas, making the trip to a center time consuming. Many of these hemophiliacs use the centers only for occasional checkups and must rely on local nonspecialist physicians and emergency rooms for care. Rita Williams, the mother of a hemophiliac, related her story of living in a rural area: "The nearest hemophilia treatment center is in Loma Linda, 65 miles away. Each trip (and there are plenty) is an 8 to 10 hour ordeal. The local hospital is closer but does not carry our product, and the staff did not feel comfortable infusing my child. I finally started using homecare. This allows me to use the local hospital, at least for emergencies." [39]

Receiving care from a physician not experienced with hemophilia can lead to errors in treatment, since the disease is rare and many doctors never treat hemophiliacs. Susan Resnik, in her book *Blood Saga*, quotes a man called "Cliff H." who has severe hemophilia, and was born in a small New Mexico town before hemophilia treatment centers were available. "Cliff" described his experience using a nonspecialist:

> There was a family doctor who was my physician during all my growing up years—he was just a family physician, not a specialist. Certainly he did not know a lot of things that he probably should have known at the time, and frankly, probably made some errors. But by the same token, he did a lot of things right. Right in the sense that he always advised me that the person who should know the most about the disease is myself. He used to give me articles he had at the time, and his counsel was, "I don't know everything that we should be doing, but we'll do the best we can." He used an awful lot of heat-

A bleeding patient receives care in a Washington, D.C., hospital; urban centers are better equipped for hemophiliacs' medical needs.

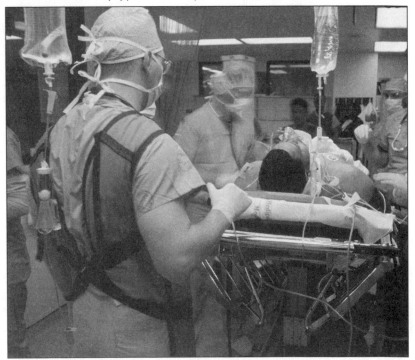

ing pads in those days that should never have been used. And that complicated a lot of factors. But for the most part all we had was whole blood, narcotics [for pain], and bed rest.[40]

Many hemophiliacs who do not live near a hemophilia treatment center keep an adequate supply of clotting factor on hand and learn home infusion.

Insurance

A final issue that must be dealt with by families of hemophiliacs is how to cover the cost of treatment. Because hemophilia is an expensive disease to treat, health insurance coverage is very important. Unfortunately, there is a downside to health insurance. In 1970, the insurance industry set a $1 million cap on lifetime coverage for an illness, meaning that is the maximum amount of money they will ever pay in a person's lifetime. Since annual treatment for an adult hemophiliac can cost between $100,000 and $200,000, it is possible to exceed the $1 million limit in five to ten years. Very few families can afford expensive hemophilia treatment without some type of financial help.

Children diagnosed with hemophilia in the first year of life will likely use their total benefits by their teen years, leaving them without insurance coverage. Children can apply for help from state-funded programs. Adults have fewer options, but may be eligible for Medicaid (a federally funded, state-operated program of medical assistance) or Social Security, which administers Medicare, a health insurance plan for people age sixty-five and over.

Hemophilia is a lifelong disease that requires the patient and family to recognize symptoms and manage treatment on an everyday basis. Patients and families with the best understanding of the disease are able to live the most normal lifestyle. Susan Cole, the mother of a child with hemophilia, has this advice. "Don't be afraid—you can handle it. Hemophilia may not be curable yet, but it's a very manageable condition."[41]

Chapter 6

The Future

RESEARCH IN GENETICS in the last part of the twentieth century promises new ways to treat hemophilia or even to cure it in the future. One of the new treatments involves cloning animals. This technology was widely reported and debated in 1997 when the first mammal was cloned. Another therapy scientists are working with is gene therapy. Since 1985, scientists have studied genes with the hope of eventually treating or curing many inherited disorders. Gene therapy is a new science, and therefore applications of the new technology will focus on relatively simple genetic defects—diseases where only one gene is at fault, like hemophilia. For hemophilia, gene therapy holds the possibility of being the very first genetic disease to be cured.

Dolly, Molly, and Polly

The first advance in future hemophilia treatment occurred in 1997, when a research laboratory in Edinburgh, Scotland, announced the successful cloning, also called nuclear transfer, of a sheep from a single cell. A clone is an exact copy of a species—in this case, an exact genetic replica of the sheep it was cloned from. The cloning of the first sheep, Dolly, proved that cloning animals could be accomplished. While Dolly's cloning had no immediate medical benefit, her birth was the first step in an effort to develop animals capable of producing milk containing human clotting factors for treating hemophilia. It took Dr. Ian Wilmut, an embryologist (a scientist who specializes in the development of an organism from conception to birth), twenty-three years to clone Dolly. Dolly was born in the summer of 1996 and made worldwide headlines the following year when her birth was announced via newspapers and scientific journals.

Dolly was conceived in a test tube by removing cells from the udders of a six-year-old female sheep. These cells were placed in a test tube and made incapable of growing or multiplying. Then DNA (genetic material) from unfertilized eggs of other female sheep was removed and combined with DNA from the udder cells. An electric current was used on each DNA combination to fuse the two together into one cell. Each fused egg then developed into an embryo, and these embryos (organisms in the earliest stage of development) were implanted into thirteen mother sheep. Only one of these sheep became pregnant and she delivered Dolly.

In late 1997, Dr. Wilmut announced the birth of new cloned sheep, named Molly and Polly. A slightly different process was used to conceive Molly and Polly than was used for Dolly. Lamb

Born in 1996, Dolly is the first successfully cloned sheep. Doctors hope to clone animals whose milk will contain clotting factors for hemophiliacs.

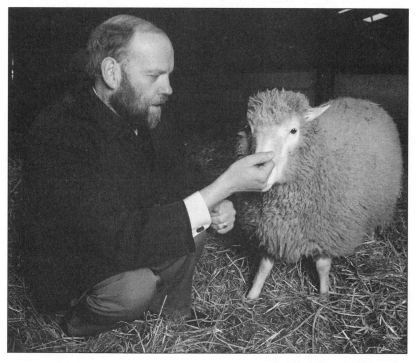

cells were injected with the human factor IX gene, so that a human blood-clotting gene became part of the sheep's DNA. Sheep cells with the DNA removed had the newly combined lamb/human clotting factor DNA added, and were allowed to grow in test tubes before being implanted into a mother sheep. Six lambs were born, and three of them had the human blood-clotting gene for factor IX. One of these lambs died, leaving Molly and Polly.

While Dolly proved that animal cloning was possible, Molly and Polly proved that animals could be used as drug-making factories. The milk produced by these sheep contains the clotting factor needed to treat people with hemophilia B. The term "pharming" has been coined to describe using animals to make pharmaceuticals (medications). Alan Colman, a research director of PPL Therapeutics, whose company sponsored Dr. Wilmut in the cloning of sheep, said, "This is the realization of our vision to produce instant flocks or herds which express high concentrations of valuable therapeutic proteins very quickly."[42]

"Pharming" Cows

Other organizations with similar goals have since cloned animals. The Red Cross, along with a Netherlands pharmaceutical company, financially backed a lab in Madison, Wisconsin, that hopes to produce an entire herd of cloned cows producing clotting factors in their milk. Dr. Leon Hoyer, director of a Red Cross laboratory in Maryland, says, "About 100 cows could make a large percentage of the world's supply of factor VIII, at much lower costs than refining it from blood."[43] Before this can happen, the Food and Drug Administration (FDA) must give approval concerning the safety and effectiveness of this method. The FDA must approve each cow producing clotting factor, just as if the cow were a laboratory. The president of the company that cloned the cows predicts it will be 2005 or 2006 before approval is obtained.

As with any new technology, there are unknowns and concerns. One of the concerns with using animals to produce medication is the possibility that animal diseases could be transmitted to humans, which means that better tests must be developed to screen animals for diseases. This problem may further delay approval of animals used to make drugs.

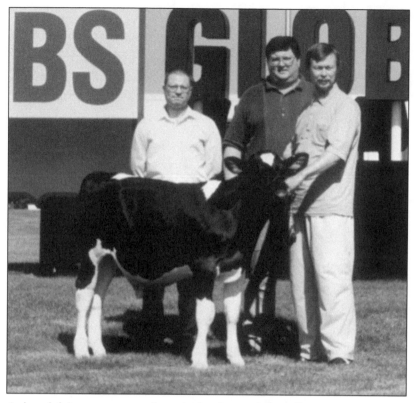

A cloned dairy cow may produce clotting factors in its milk.

A second concern with cloning centers on the fear that the next step after cloning animals is cloning humans, which worries many people. One ethical problem is that cloned humans could be used to create a race of people in a discriminatory fashion, eliminating traits seen as undesirable and only cloning people with desirable characteristics. Another concern is that cloned individuals might come into life with preconceived expectations placed on them, such as the expectation to possess great athletic ability or high intelligence. Finally, legal issues center on who has legal responsibility for a clone: Without biological parents, who would raise a cloned child? Also, there are fears that cloning could be done without the consent of the person being cloned, which violates the principle in medicine of a person giving informed consent before a procedure is performed.

Genes Revisited

While sheep and cows were cloned to make drugs, other scientists were working on finding a cure for hemophilia by attempting gene therapy—treating diseases by replacing defective genes in the body. To understand gene therapy, it is necessary to understand DNA, genes, and chromosomes and their relationship to cells.

The human body is composed of trillions of cells. In each cell nucleus of a human are twenty-three pairs of chromosomes, half of each pair inherited from the mother and half from the father. DNA (deoxyribonucleic acid) is composed of various chemicals, which make up the structure of a chromosome. Each cell has a six-foot thread of DNA folded up to fit the microscopic space. Genes are segments of DNA that instruct a cell about its job. There are thirty thousand to forty thousand genes in the human genome, which is all the genetic material making up a species contained in each cell. Each species—humans, dogs, even worms—has a different genome. Rick Weiss, a science writer for the *Washington Post*, explained the complexity of the human genome: "It [the human genome] can be thought of as a huge encyclopedia that is written as a single enormously long sentence of 3.1 billion letters, with virtually no punctuation along the way. . . . This six-foot long rambling molecular sentence is folded inside almost every one of the body's 100 trillion cells. Genes are individual portions of the run-on text, ranging in size from about 1,000 to 100,000 letters."[44]

The National Health Museum compares the size of cells, chromosomes, and genes to features on a map of the earth. If a cell is compared to the earth, then chromosomes could be compared to a country, and genes to a city. In hemophilia, the gene that instructs the body to make clotting factors VIII or IX is located near the tip of one of the X chromosomes, whose function is to determine sex.

Gene Therapy

While cloning is designed to create an exact replica of an animal, gene therapy is a medical treatment to repair genes or replace missing or nonfunctional genes. Research is currently progressing in gene therapy with the hope of curing some genetic disorders, including hemophilia. This means placing normal factor VIII or IX genes into cells so a person with one of these bleeding problems would begin producing clotting factor on his own. In the immediate future, the hope is to raise levels of clotting factor for extended periods of time, so that hemophiliacs will no longer require frequent doses of factor replacement. The final goal is to cure hemophilia by discovering a way for replacement genes to live permanently in the body and not be destroyed inside dying cells.

There are two methods for placing genes inside cells. One method is called in vivo and means the transfer of genes occurs inside the patient. An example of a clinical trial using the in vivo method involves modifying a virus called a retrovirus so it cannot replicate (make a copy of itself), then placing a gene for factor VIII

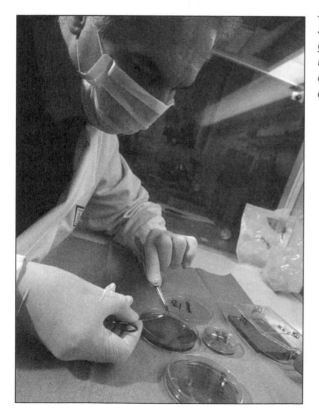

A scientist performs gene therapy in hopes of finding a cure for AIDS and other diseases.

inside it and transferring this gene directly to the patient. In ex vivo, the transfer of genes occurs outside the patient, and then the modified gene is placed inside the body. An example of ex vivo is removing cells from a patient by surgery, growing them in culture, modifying them, and then surgically returning them to the patient. This method is more time consuming than in vivo.

To transfer a gene, it is necessary to use a vector, which is anything capable of transporting the gene into the cell. Liposomes, which are fat molecules, have been used as vectors. However, the most common type of vector is a virus. Viruses require cells to survive, so they are good at finding and delivering genes to cells. The problem, of course, with viruses is that most of them cause disease, so modification of the virus is accomplished by removing the parts that allow it to multiply to the point where sickness occurs. Another problem is that viruses are very small, and one virus may not be able to carry a large gene, such as the factor VIII gene. Some of the viruses used are the adenovirus that produces the common cold; a lentivirus, which is an AIDS-like virus; a retrovirus; and a virus called adeno-associated virus (AAV). This last virus has been used in some of the more successful gene therapy trials because it is not known to cause human disease and does not cause the body to reject it by signaling the immune system. Other researchers favor the adenovirus because it is eight times larger than the adeno-associated virus and can carry larger genes.

Choosing a Target

Once the gene is modified and inserted in a vector, researchers must decide on a target cell in the patient's body. One of the target cells that is used for hemophilia patients is a liver cell, because that is where clotting factor is normally produced. Muscle or skin cells have also been used, particularly if the person has liver disease. In choosing target cells, scientists consider the life span of the cell, how easy the cell is to reach, and how rapidly the cell multiplies, because more rapidly dividing cells ensure longer-lasting treatment. Gene therapy is delivered to a patient by intravenous injection, by intramuscular injection, or by surgical implantation of the gene.

Another consideration about where to implant modified genes concerns whether to place them in somatic (body) cells or put them in germ (egg and sperm) cells. Putting new genes into body cells has the desired effect of changing the cell so it functions correctly but doesn't transmit the change to future generations. Adding the altered gene to a germ cell would pass the change to the person's offspring. At present, germ line therapy is not approved for use by the government. Kevin Kelley, in writing about gene therapy in a hemophilia newsletter, says, "Gene therapy is complex: it involves adding DNA to a patient's cells, perhaps even altering some of the patient's own DNA. Once made, these changes could be extremely difficult or impossible to reverse." [45]

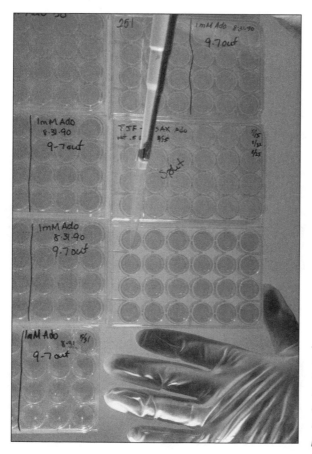

Marked culture dishes help a researcher identify and replace harmful genes in a patient's DNA.

Progress and Setbacks in Gene Therapy

In 1999, Dr. Katherine High, a hematologist at the Children's Hospital of Philadelphia, announced that gene therapy had achieved long-term improvement in naturally occurring hemophilia in dogs. The dog's level of clotting factor was raised to 4 to 12 percent of normal, which is enough to prevent the need for daily factor replacement. Dr. High used the adeno-associated virus (AAV) as the vector to deliver the gene. Once success with dogs was documented, she used the treatment on adult patients with hemophilia B. The gene was given to patients by intramuscular injection into leg and arm muscles.

The most devastating setback in gene therapy occurred in September of 1999 with the death of eighteen-year-old Jesse Gelsinger, who was receiving gene therapy with an adenovirus vector for a rare liver disease. The virus caused a flulike illness, which is thought to have contributed to his death. The FDA temporarily halted all gene therapy trials in eight labs until scientists demonstrated better monitoring of studies.

The first success in gene therapy for people with hemophilia A was reported in the June 7, 2001, issue of the *New England Journal of Medicine*. In this experiment a skin cell from a severe type A hemophiliac was used instead of the viral vectors previously used to transfer the gene. DNA containing factor VIII was added to the skin cell. This single cell was replicated until there were more than one hundred million cells, which were then injected into fat in six patients' abdomens. Four of the six patients showed great improvement in clotting ability, and the results lasted three months.

Gene therapy is not as simple a technique as was once imagined. Many scientists believed that gene therapy would cure hemophilia by the year 2000. It is now estimated that it may take until the year 2010 for an FDA-approved therapy to become available to hemophiliacs. W. French Anderson, a gene therapy pioneer, says, "What it comes down to is that gene therapy, although it sounds simple, is like putting a man on the moon. It's an incredibly complex endeavor." [46]

Exploring Other Ways to Help Hemophiliacs

In 2000, research was reported that used a different approach to treating hemophilia. This experiment, tried on rhesus monkeys, used a porous (capable of being penetrated) chamber implanted in the abdomen that continuously converts factor VII into a factor that allows blood to clot without the missing factors VIII or IX. This research effectively bypasses the need to give clotting factors VIII or IX intravenously, and would allow the hemophiliac access to a supply of clotting factor manufactured by his own body. The procedure would require surgery to implant the chamber into the abdomen. Scientists expect it to be effective for both types of hemophilia. Clinical testing on humans with hemophilia will be necessary before the device is available.

Another research study attempting to correct the genetic defect in hemophilia was reported in February 2002 at a children's hospital in Germany. In this experiment, scientists transferred healthy clotting factor genes into unborn mice. The treatment proved successful because production of clotting factors continued for several months past birth. Viruses were used to transfer human clotting factor IX into the unborn mice. Researchers think an advantage of performing gene transfer before birth is the baby's immature immune system, which makes it less likely to form antibodies against the clotting factors. The therapy has not been attempted on unborn human babies.

Finally, the American Red Cross has launched a program to support care in underdeveloped countries where hemophiliacs receive little or no treatment. This multimillion-dollar project, called Care 2000, provides resources that will improve care for hemophiliacs around the world. Part of this project includes educating health care providers, sponsoring research in genetics, and providing products to hemophilia communities in need.

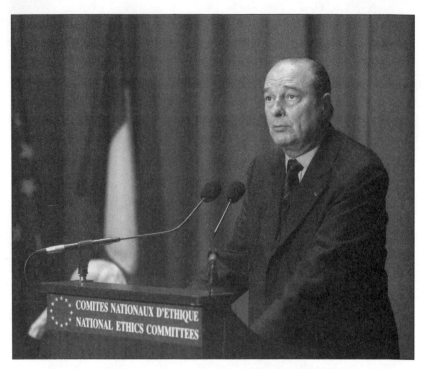

New advances in cloning and genetic research prompts ethical debate at world conferences like the National Ethics Committees (pictured).

The last fifteen years has provided some exciting advances in treatment for hemophilia. Yet, much of the research is in the early stages. Doubts exist about the ethics of cloning, especially the possibility that cloning animals for medical treatment will evolve into cloning humans for reasons less worthy. Many are concerned about gene therapy and the long-term effects on the body. As one anonymous mother said when faced with the possibility that gene therapy might soon be an option for her hemophiliac son, "My child is doing fine on his factor concentrate. I would rather wait 15 years after its approval to see how well gene therapy will work."[47] Despite her concerns, most scientists believe that a safe cure for hemophilia will occur. The question is not whether it will occur, but when.

Notes

Introduction: Hemophilia—An Ancient Disease with a Promising Future

1. Quoted in Hemophilia Galaxy "Hemophilia Treatment: Where We've Been and Where We're Going," 2002. www.hemophiliagalaxy.com.

Chapter 1: Understanding Hemophilia

2. Quoted in Laureen Kelley, *Raising a Child with Hemophilia*. 3d. ed. King of Prussia, PA: Aventis Behring L.L.C., 1999, p. 27.
3. Quoted in Kelley, *Raising a Child*, p. 2.
4. Peter M. Green, "This Bad Blood," *The Lancet*, December 2001, p. S34.
5. Quoted in Kelley, *Raising a Child*, p. 93.
6. Quoted in Hemophilia Galaxy, "Profiles: Baxter Therapies and Services," 2002. www.hemophiliagalaxy.com.
7. Quoted in Kelley, *Raising a Child*, p. 24.
8. Quoted in Kelley, *Raising a Child*, p. 45.
9. Green, "This Bad Blood," p. S34.

Chapter 2: Hemophilia Throughout History

10. Quoted in Hemophilia Galaxy, "Five Key People in Hemophilia History," 2002. www.hemophiliagalaxy.com.
11. Quoted in Douglas Starr, *Blood: An Epic History of Medicine and Commerce*. New York: Alfred A. Knopf, 1998, p. 46.
12. Quoted in Hemophilia Galaxy, "Hemophilia Treatment."
13. Quoted in Susan Resnik, *Blood Saga: Hemophilia, AIDS, and the Survival of a Community*. Berkeley: University of California Press, 1999, p. 16.
14. Quoted in Resnik, *Blood Saga*, p. 16.

15. Quoted in Resnik, *Blood Saga*, p. 16.

16. Quoted in Hemophilia Galaxy, "First Recombinant Factor VIII Patient Infuses Hemophilia Community with Hope," 2002. www.hemophiliagalaxy.com.

17. Quoted in Hemophilia Galaxy, "First Recombinant Factor VIII Patient."

18. Quoted in Hemophilia Galaxy, "Hemophilia Treatment."

Chapter 3: Diagnosis and Treatment

19. Quoted in Hemophilia Galaxy, "Take a Journey into Genetics to Understand Hemophilia Better," 2002. www.hemophilia galaxy.com.

20. Quoted in Fairfield University: Hemophilia, "My Factor Story," June 27, 2000. www.faculty.fairfield.edu.

21. Quoted in Hemophilia Galaxy, "Teenagers Have Their Say About Living with Hemophilia," 2002. www.hemophilia galaxy.com.

22. Quoted in Hemophilia Galaxy, "We're Working for You, Creighton Peterson!" 2002. www.hemophiliagalaxy.com.

23. Quoted in Hemophilia Galaxy, "Joint Damage, Let's Get Physical," 2002. www.hemophiliagalaxy.com.

24. Quoted in Kelley, *Raising a Child*, p.13.

25. Quoted in Hemophilia Galaxy, "'The Big Stick' Yields Big Results," 2002. www.hemophiliagalaxy.com.

Chapter 4: Complications

26. Quoted in "Ryan White's Testimony before the President's Commission." www.geocities.com.

27. Quoted in Resnick, *Blood Saga*, p. 19.

28. Quoted in Kelley, *Raising a Child*, p. 280.

29. Quoted in Hemophilia Access, Inc., "Uncommon Bleeds." www.hemophiliaccess.com.

30. Quoted in FAMOHIO, Inc., "Definitions," November 19, 1997. www.famohio.org.

31. Quoted in "Ryan White's Testimony."

32. Quoted in John Donnelly, "(MH) Hemophilia, Ricky, AIDS, 'It Didn't Need to Happen,'" December 15, 1992. www.aegis.com.

33. Quoted in Liz Doup, "Herald Link," *Miami Herald*, November 18, 1997. www.aegis.com.

Chapter 5: Living with Hemophilia—An Accident Waiting to Happen

34. Quoted in Hemophilia Galaxy, "Surviving the Turbulent Teens," 2002. www.hemophiliagalaxy.com.
35. Quoted in Kelley, *Raising a Child*, p. 335.
36. Quoted in Hemophilia Galaxy, "Take a Journey into Genetics."
37. Quoted in Kelley, *Raising a Child*, p. 137.
38. Quoted in Kelley, *Raising a Child*, p. 223.
39. Quoted in Kelley, *Raising a Child*, p. 268.
40. Quoted in Resnik, *Blood Saga*, pp. 28, 29.
41. Quoted in Hemophilia Galaxy, "Profiles: Baxter Therapies and Services."

Chapter 6: The Future

42. Quoted in Barry Bittman, M.D., "Hello Dolly: Or Is It Polly?" 1998–1999. www.mind-body.org.
43. Quoted in Stuart F. Brown, "From Cow's Milk to Medicine Chest," *Fortune*, New York, September 4, 2000, pp. 52–56.
44. Rick Weiss, "For DNA, a Defining Moment," *Washington Post*, May 23, 2000, p. A01.
45. Kevin Kelley, "The Hope and Hype of Hemophilia Gene Therapy," *Parent Exchange Newsletter*, February 1999. www.kelleycom.com.
46. Quoted in Liza Jane Maltin, "For Gene Therapy, It Was a Very Good Year," WebMD, December 29, 2000. http://my.webmd.com.
47. Quoted in Kelley, "The Hope and Hype of Hemophilia Gene Therapy."

Glossary

AIDS (acquired immune deficiency syndrome): The disease that occurs when a person is infected with HIV. It severely affects a person's ability to fight off infections by destroying cells in the immune system.

amniocentesis: A procedure in which amniotic fluid, which surrounds an infant in the uterus, is sampled to detect genetic diseases.

arthropathy: Any disease affecting a joint.

carrier: A person who is capable of infecting others with a disease without becoming sick themselves.

chorionic villus sampling: A method of sampling placental tissue to diagnose genetic illnesses before birth.

chromosomes: Found inside cells and made up of genes. Humans have forty-six chromosomes, half from the mother and half from the father.

circumcision: A minor surgical procedure performed on newborn males to remove the foreskin of the penis. It can be performed for religious or medical reasons.

cloning: A process for producing a genetically identical cell or organism.

clotting cascade (also called coagulation cascade): A series of steps in blood clotting where various clotting factors, designated by roman numerals, each stimulate the next clotting factor to produce a final solid blood clot.

cryoprecipitate: The product formed from freezing human plasma so it separates into layers. The bottom layer is rich in

91

human clotting factor VIII and can be administered to hemophiliacs to aid blood clotting.

dominant trait: An inherited trait capable of expressing itself in offspring with only one defective gene inherited from a parent.

embryo: Any organism in a very early stage of development. An embryo can describe anything from a few cells to early organ development.

factor assay (also called coagulating factors concentration or blood-clotting factors): A blood test that measures the quantity of any of the blood-clotting factors in a person's blood, such as factor VIII or factor IX.

factor VIII: The clotting factor missing in classic hemophilia, or hemophilia A.

factor IX: The clotting factor missing in hemophilia B, also known as Christmas disease.

FDA (Food and Drug Administration): A federal agency that regulates the manufacture of foods, drugs, and cosmetics to prevent the sale or use of dangerous products.

gene: A unit of heredity located on a chromosome inside a cell. Each gene codes for a different characteristic.

gene therapy: Treating genetic diseases by transferring healthy genes into a person's body.

hemarthrosis: Bleeding into a joint.

hematologist: A physician specializing in diseases of the blood and immune system.

hepatitis: An inflammation of the liver.

HIV (human immunodeficiency virus): The virus causing AIDS. It affects a person's ability to withstand infections and may take up to ten years to fully develop into disease.

hormone: A chemical produced by the body whose function is to regulate the activity of another part of the body. Most hormones circulate in the blood.

immune tolerance therapy: A treatment for overcoming inhibitors some hemophiliacs develop to infused clotting factors. The therapy consists of high doses of clotting factors given on a frequent basis to get the body accustomed to the needed treatment.

inhibitors: In hemophilia, an inhibitor is a reaction by the body against infused clotting factors, rendering them ineffective.

Medicaid: A federally funded, state-operated program to help low-income families pay for medical care.

Medicare: A U.S. federally funded health insurance program for people over sixty-five.

mutation: An unusual change in a gene that prevents it from performing its normal function. Mutations can be triggered by chemicals or radiation and can occur spontaneously.

nuclear transfer: Another name for the process involved in cloning.

pharming: A coined word meaning cloning animals capable of producing medications (pharmaceuticals).

plasma: The clear, liquid part of blood where clotting factors circulate.

prophylaxis (prebleed treatment): In hemophilia, prophylaxis refers to preventing bleeding by administering clotting factors on a schedule prior to any bleeding episodes.

recessive trait: An inherited trait that requires two defective genes, one from each parent, before the trait is seen in offspring.

recombinant DNA: A DNA molecule in which genes have been artificially rearranged.

replication: The duplication of the genetic material (DNA) in a cell to make an exact copy. The DNA splits into two strands and takes on new chemicals to make a replica of itself.

synovium: A membrane around a joint secreting a lubricating fluid.

target cell: A cell chosen for the new home of the gene being transferred.

target joint: Any joint that bleeds frequently in a hemophiliac. This joint is most likely to develop arthritis.

vector: A vehicle to carry genes into human cells in gene therapy. Commonly used vectors are viruses rendered incapable of causing disease.

For Further Reading

Books

Larry Gonick and Mark Wheelis, *The Cartoon Guide to Genetics*. New York: Harper Collins, 1991. While designed for older students, this book goes step by step into genetics, DNA, and recombinant DNA. Because it is several years old, some of the newer technologies like gene therapy and cloning are not included; however, it is very well done. Illustrations include talking peas, opinionated fruit flies, and dancing scientists.

Jacqueline L. Harris, *Bodies in Crisis: Hereditary Diseases*. New York: Twenty-First Century Books, 1993. This is an age-appropriate book explaining chromosomes and genes and how they cause disease. It includes a chapter on outside agents and their effect on hereditary diseases. There is a limited discussion of hemophilia, and the book includes good pictures and drawings of chromosomes and patterns of inheritance.

Kelly Huegal and Elizabeth Verdick, *Young People and Chronic Illness: True Stories, Help, and Hope*. Minneapolis, MN: Free Spirit Publications, 1998. True stories of children with chronic illnesses as they talk about their diseases. Hemophilia is one of the illnesses discussed.

Chris Oyler, *Go Toward the Light*. New York: Harper and Row, 1988. The true story of Ben Oyler, a young boy with hemophilia, who contracted AIDS at age seven from a blood transfusion treatment for his hemophilia. Ben died from AIDS.

Charlotte Zeepvat, *Prince Leopold: The Untold Story of Queen Victoria's Youngest Son*. London: Sutton Publishing, 2000. A 224-page biography of Prince Leopold, a hemophiliac and the son of Queen Victoria of England. He was the first famous person recognized with hemophilia, and details of his illness were published in a British medical journal.

Free Videos on Hemophilia

Inside a Bleeding Joint
This free video is for children and is narrated by a child. It includes an explanation of hemophilia, how joints work, and what happens when joint bleeding occurs.

Bayer Corporation
Pharmaceutical Division
400 Morgan Road
West Haven, CT 06516-4175

Learning About Hemophilia
A twenty-four-minute video covering hemophilia, levels of severity, genetics, care, and factor replacement. Comes with a booklet.

Therapeutic Services
1127 Bryn Mawr Avenue
Redlands, CA 92374

Self-Infusion: Gateway to Independence
This is a twenty-minute video plus a book that teaches hemophiliacs how to self-infuse clotting factors.

Anne Marie Pierce
Centeon
1020 First Avenue
King of Prussia, PA
19406-1310

Organizations to Contact

The Centers for Disease Control and Prevention (CDC)
1600 Clifton Road
Atlanta, GA 30333
(404) 639-3925
http://www.cdc.gov
The CDC's main job is to provide surveillance and investigations for epidemics. However, the U.S. Congress has mandated a National Hemophilia Program, and the CDC has undertaken the mission of reducing or preventing complications of hemophilia and other bleeding disorders.

Coalition for Hemophilia B, Inc.
712 Fifth Avenue, 43rd Floor
New York, NY 10019
(212) 554-6823
Fax:(212) 554-6906
E-mail: cfb@web-depot.com
The parents of a child with hemophilia B started this organization. The goal is to support research, provide education, and network with pharmaceutical companies.

COTT: The Committee of Ten Thousand
906 D Street, NE
Washington, DC 20002
(800) 230-9797
The committee advocates for families and patients with clotting disorders who are infected with HIV/AIDS. It is named for the estimated ten thousand hemophiliacs in the United States infected with HIV/AIDS through use of contaminated blood products.

L. A. Kelley Communications, Inc.
68 East Main Street
Suite 102
Georgetown, MA 01833
(800) 249-7977
(978) 352-7657
Fax: (978) 352-6254
E-mail: laurie@kelleycom.com
http://www.kelleycom.com
Laureen Kelley, the mother of a child with hemophilia, founded this private organization. Mrs. Kelley has written and illustrated several age-appropriate educational books and booklets about hemophilia, which are free on request. Other services offered include newsletters, workshops, and educational meetings, as well as family support.

The National Hemophilia Foundation (NHF)
116 West 32nd Street, 11th Floor
New York, NY 10001
(800) 42-HANDI
(212) 328-3700
Fax: (212) 328-3799
E-mail: info@hemophilia.org
http://www.hemophilia.org
The NHF is dedicated to hemophilia education and research. HANDI is the name of its branch providing literature and general information. The organization as a whole develops educational materials, raises funds, promotes research, and serves as a communication center for issues related to hemophilia. They sponsor forty-two hemophilia chapters throughout the United States.

World Federation of Hemophilia (WFH)
1425 René; LeVesque Boulevard West
Suite 1010
Montreal, Quebec, Canada H3G IT7
(514) 875-7944
E-mail: wfh@wfh.org
http://www.wfh.org
This international organization offers a wide range of programs related to bleeding disorders. Its scope is worldwide, promoting information exchange between countries.

Works Consulted

Books

Laureen A. Kelley, *Alexis, the Prince Who Had Hemophilia*. King of Prussia, PA: Aventis Behring, L.L.C., 2001. An illustrated biography of Alexis, the son of Alexandra and Nicholas of Russia. It details his childhood as a hemophiliac and the effect of the disease on his family and the history of his country. The book includes a family tree showing the lines of transmission of hemophilia in the royal families of Europe.

Laureen A. Kelley, *Raising a Child with Hemophilia*. (3rd). King of Prussia, PA: Aventis Behring L.L.C., 1999. This is a comprehensive book written as a guide for parents of a hemophiliac. It includes everything from an explanation of the disease to treatment and handling everyday problems. The book liberally quotes both parents and hemophiliacs about their experiences.

Kathleen Pagana and Timothy J. Pagana, *Mosby's Diagnostic and Laboratory Test Reference*. 5th ed. St. Louis, MO: Mosby, 2001. A reference source for medical professionals listing various diagnostic and laboratory tests, explaining how they are performed, and including preparation for the tests with normal results.

Roy Porter, *The Greatest Benefit to Mankind*. New York: W. W. Norton, 1997. Outlines the medical history of the world from antiquity to the end of the twentieth century. The book has chapters on surgery, psychiatry, public medicine, and tropical and world diseases, as well as medicine related to various cultures.

Susan Resnik, *Blood Saga: Hemophilia, AIDS, and the Survival of a Community*. Berkeley: University of California Press, 1999. This book details the early days of hemophilia followed by the effect of the HIV-contaminated blood supply on the hemophilia community. It is a detailed and well-researched book.

Douglas Starr, *Blood: An Epic History of Medicine and Commerce*. New York: Alfred A. Knopf, 1998. The book contains a history of blood's medical uses from the past to the present. It includes everything from ancient bloodletting practices to the AIDS crisis of the 1980s.

Periodicals

Blood Weekly, "Prenatal Gene Transfer Proposed for Treating Hemophilia, Other Diseases," February 14, 2002.

Brian Bergstein, "Work Shows Gene Healing's Promise," *Houston Chronicle*, December 10, 2000.

Stuart F. Brown, "From Cow's Milk to Medicine Chest," *Fortune*, New York, September 4, 2000.

Peter M. Green, "This Bad Blood," *The Lancet*, December 2001.

Doug Ireland, "Remember Ricky Ray," *New Nation, New York*, November 15, 1999.

Peter Jones, M.D., "Growing Up with Hemophilia: Four Articles on Childhood," a publication of the Hemophilia Treatment Center, Los Angeles, California, 1994.

Amy Slugg Moore, "Apparatus Holds Promise for Hemophiliacs," *RN*, June 2000.

Judy Schaefer, "Ethical Dilemmas in the Pediatric Hemophilia Community," *Pediatric Nursing*, 1999.

New Scientist, "Hemophilia Hope: Gene Therapy Provides Improvement for Patients," December 16, 2000.

Rick Weiss, "For DNA, a Defining Moment," *Washington Post*, May 23, 2000.

Internet Sources

Barry Bittman, M.D., "Hello Dolly: Or Is It Polly?" 1998–1999. www.mind-body.org.

John Donnelly, "(MH) Hemophilia, Ricky, AIDS, 'It Didn't Need to Happen,'" *Miami Herald,* December 15, 1992. www.aegis.com.

Fairfield University, "My Factor Story," June 27, 2000. www.faculty.fairfield.edu.

Geocities, "Ryan White's Testimony before the President's Commission." www.geocities.com.

Hemophilia Access, Inc., "Uncommon Bleeds." www. hemophiliaccess.com.

Hemophilia Galaxy, 'The Big Stick' Yields Big Results," 2002. www.hemophiliagalaxy.com.

————, "First Recombinant Factor VIII Patient Infuses Hemophilia Community with Hope," 2002.

————, "Five Key People in Hemophilia History," 2002.

————, "Hemophilia Treatment: Where We've Been and Where We're Going," 2002.

————, "Joint Damage: Let's Get Physical," 2002.

————, Profiles: Baxter Therapies and Services, 2002.

————, "Surviving the Turbulent Teens," 2002.

————, "Take a Journey into Genetics to Understand Hemophilia Better," 2002.

————, "Teenagers Have Their Say About Living with Hemophilia," 2002.

————, "We're Working for You, Creighton Peterson!" 2002.

Kevin C. Kelley, "The Hope and Hype of Hemophilia Gene Therapy," *Parent Exchange Newsletter,* February 1999. www.kelleycom.com.

Liza Jane Maltin, "For Gene Therapy, It Was a Very Good Year," *WebMD,* December 29, 2000. http://my.webmd.com.

Websites

American Medical Association's Council on Ethical and Judicial Affairs (www.ama-assn.org). This is the official website of the American Medical Association representing medical doctors across the United States. The Council on Ethical and Judicial Affairs, a committee of the AMA, maintains and updates the AMA Code of Medical Ethics including positions on current issues like cloning.

American Red Cross (www.redcross.org). The Red Cross provides health and safety services to the American public including HIV/AIDS education. They also provide support to underdeveloped countries where hemophiliacs receive little or no care, sponsor research in genetics, and educate health care providers about hemophilia.

Pediatric Database (www.icondata.com). The site contains comprehensive data with information on both rare and common pediatric conditions.

United States Department of Health and Human Services (www.os.dhhs.gov). The Department of Health and Human Services is the government's main agency to protect the health of all Americans. The department sponsors 300 programs including financial assistance to low-income families, information on drug safety, research projects, and handles Medicare claims. One of the subgroups is the National Heart, Lung, and Blood Institute, which offers information on blood-related disorders like hemophilia. Their website is www.nhlbi.nih.gov.

Index

Picture Credits

About the Author

Beverly Britton is a registered nurse with a diploma in nursing from St. Luke's Hospital, Kansas City, Missouri; a bachelor's degree in nursing from the University of Texas Health Science Center in Houston; and a master's in nursing from Texas Woman's University. In addition to working in numerous clinical nursing positions, she was a professor of nursing at North Harris Montgomery Community College in Houston for twenty years. She lives in The Woodlands, Texas, with her husband, Bob, and two dogs, Spike and Buttercup.